7 SYSTEMS PLAN

Proven Steps
to Amazing Health Transformations
and Lasting Weight Loss

BY DR. PAT LUSE

AUTHOR
ACADEMY elite

One part common sense, one part scientific genius, this book treats the underlying root causes of being out of shape, not just the visible symptoms of obesity. Should be mandatory reading for everyone over the age of 12.

—Angie Bullock

Dr. Pat Luse gets it. For those of us who have struggled with unexplained weight issues for years, we finally have someone who understands that our body is not functioning correctly. When I heard Dr. Pat speak a year ago, I couldn't wait to buy his book and read it. As I did, so much of his observations, scientific research, and process made sense. And as I read it, I kept saying, "Thank you for getting the struggle." And thank you for working hard to find the solution for your patients and me.

—Kirsten Samuel

I've run around in holistic wellness circles for years, but I learned so much reading this book! It clearly summarizes an amazing amount of information in a highly readable and even entertaining format. It's chock-full of helpful resources.

— Abigail Young

I must confess when I first saw this book, I said to myself, "I can't read another one!" I was so wrong! This is not just another quick fix. This is a FIX! Dr. Luse shows you the steps to take so that your body will heal each System. Don't wait like I did. Buy it now!

—Anita McLaurin

In *7 Systems Plan*, Dr. Pat Luse walks you through the Systems of the body and how they contribute to health. He also helps you diagnose which systems might be failing you and what you can do about it. This book is for you if you're struggling with weight gain, fatigue, brain fog, IBS, high blood pressure, diabetes, etc. Dr. Luse is very methodical and will get you moving toward better health quickly.

—Allan Misner

I have been fortunate to have experienced the 7 Systems Plan through Dr. Luse's local clinic. I have lost over 65 pounds and have kept it off. More importantly, however, I have regained my health. Though I have had local support, I have found this book to be invaluable to my continuing success. This book not only explains WHAT to do but also WHY. It has a great appendix which lays out resources for each chapter such as shopping lists, journal sample, success plan, etc. It is easy to comprehend, and I take it everywhere that I may have a few minutes to read—It's like having a life coach in my pocket.

Anyone who struggles with food needs the research-based information this book provides. And once you are armed with the knowledge, it is easier to make the healthy decision. For example, just when I think I need a snack before bed, I'm reminded what that does to my mitochondria and how that sabotages my health.

This book is for ANYONE who wants to improve their health, whether you have 5 or 150 pounds to lose.

—kickboxerjd

Dropped 50 pounds, size 16 to 8, and lowered cholesterol 80 points in 6 months!

- Reversed fatty liver disease—liver numbers returned to normal!
- Feeling very energetic and joint pain minimal now!
- My personal trainer said I was stronger than four years ago.

These are the results I experienced with the 7 Systems Plan! I had tried to lose weight and had many ups and downs and then ups in the past. I just couldn't get and keep the weight off until following this plan. I had given up and decided being fat was the new normal. I was amazed it really made such a difference after other diet plans could not. My doctors were all surprised. I have kept the weight off one year now, and I'm confident I can keep it off for good and head off an early grave with the tools Dr. Luse provides. Friends who haven't seen me in a while are amazed at the transformation and are asking for the book and website!

—Rhonda Miller

Great read. Thought-provoking look at how the body is made of Systems and how they all work together for optimum health. Many ideas you can easily implement and get started down a path to a healthier you.

— Chellie

A Word from My Patients

"I initially started this program to lose the weight that I had gained over the past three years. But it has turned into so much more than that for me. I always knew how to lose weight and what I should be eating. I struggled with the maintenance because I'd usually revert to my former ways of eating. Other programs often leave out the why, and that's what makes the 7 Systems Plan different.

"It isn't all about the weight loss for me now—it's about leading a healthy lifestyle. Understanding what happens in my body's Systems when I turn to sugar has made such an impact on me that I will not do that to myself ever again. My health is my primary focus—the weight loss is a side effect. I now have the tools, knowledge, and support to make this a lasting lifestyle. At age 51, I have never felt better."

—Jo Dee Weltz

"Prior to going through the program with Dr. Luse ... as a type 1 diabetic, I used on average over 100 units of insulin daily. I have cut my insulin by more than 50%. When I first started going through the 7 Systems Plan, I ate meals with an inhaler because of severe allergies. I no longer eat with an inhaler. I lost a total of 82 pounds, and I have kept the weight off for four years. I now have much more energy and am able to move and enjoy life once again. Thank you, Dr. Luse, for giving me my health back."

—Lucinda Mason

"A few years ago, Dr. Pat Luse looked at my lab work and said, "You're headed for a train wreck." He gave me suggestions, but due to my out-of-control food addiction, I walked away and went back to my old eating habits, which wreaked havoc with my diabetes.

"Sure enough, two years later I became deathly ill. I was sent by ambulance to the hospital where I would spend the next 45 days. In addition to being diagnosed with pancreatitis, my triglycerides soared to 3,500, my blood sugars to 1,000, my kidneys were shutting down, and my stomach was literally rotting. I was put into ICU and heavily sedated. A ventilator and feeding tube kept me alive while my body fought for life. The doctors told my family, "Sheila will die without surgery, and we don't think she will live through surgery. Tell her good-bye." Medically speaking, I should have died, but God had another plan.

"After that, I read a lot about healthy fats and intermittent fasting, but due to my food addiction, I couldn't put it all together and continued to eat way too much. It wasn't until I read *7 Systems Plan* that the pieces and missing links started coming together. As I began applying the principles in *7 Systems Plan*, the weight started coming off. I drastically reduced insulin, sleep much better (so I wake up feeling rested), and haven't needed to take Rolaids. I also do not need to get up and use the bathroom in the night even though I am drinking more water, to say nothing of the improved energy and positive attitude toward life again. Instead of sitting around most of the day, I am getting lots of things done. *7 Systems Plan* has given me hope and freedom from the constant war within me regarding food."

—Sheila Dixon

"I became really sick around the holidays three years ago and continued to get worse over the next nine months. Every joint in my body was inflamed and very painful. I could barely walk or move. I am self-employed and was unable to work. Washing my hands brought tears to my eyes. I thought my fingers would just break off from the force of the water.

"I was treated for Lyme disease and rheumatoid arthritis, and then was told that I had some kind of 'inflammatory process' that couldn't be diagnosed. I either had to have help or lean on the walls to get to the bathroom. It was a nightmare. I was going downhill fast.

"Before completely giving up, I decided to go see Dr. Luse. He said he thought he could help me feel an improvement in just 10 days. I thought he didn't know what he was dealing with. I decided it was my last attempt to salvage myself. I went home that day with the 7 Systems Plan.

"After five days, I realized I was walking on my own to the bathroom. I felt a thrill of excitement and hoped it wasn't a dream. I went to my computer and told Dr. Pat Luse how I had moved and walked unaided, and I thanked him from the bottom of my heart.

"With Dr. Pat Luse's guidance, I have not only regained my health, but I have also continuously improved it. At the start, I didn't care about anything but hanging onto my life! In the process, I also lost 20 pounds. My body and mind feel better than they have in years. Every time I tell this story, I choke up. I can't adequately put into words my heartfelt gratitude. Thank you, Dr. Luse."

—Nancy Lorenzen

"Dr. Pat Luse has devoted his life to studying natural health. He has researched products and theories and helped his patients survive and even thrive. Dr. Pat has given my husband, Doug, and me the tools to maintain a healthy weight, eat wisely, exercise efficiently, detoxify our bodies, deal with stress, and get better sleep. We have lost weight and kept it off. As a result of the weight loss, Doug is no longer diabetic, and he was able to quit taking diabetic medications altogether.

"Before following Dr. Pat's health plan, Doug would catch any little 'bug' that was going around. Now that he starts his day with the recommended 'medical food' and a simple vitamin regimen, he is rarely bothered by the colds and flu that used to plague him continuously.

"We are so happy that we were able to get this help. We made lifestyle changes that have become routine. Our level of health is greatly improved, and we have peace of mind knowing that we are minimizing illness and disability in order to age gracefully and enjoy the best possible health. Dr. Pat's training empowers people to understand what it takes to be healthy and gives them the tools to get there."

—Shirley & Doug Patrick

"Dr. Luse's book, *7 Systems Plan*, will forever change your understanding of how nutrition and exercise affect your life. I had been on numerous diets and exercise plans and had spent thousands of dollars to lose weight only to gain the pounds back and fall into my old habits. My body was not only overweight, but I was in poor health and very close to being diabetic. I had already vowed to never pay anyone another dollar to help me lose weight. But I decided to take one more risk with Dr. Luse's plan. Finally!

"I learned how my body interacts with food. I learned the connection between nutrition and exercise, which build a metabolism that doesn't struggle to maintain itself. There's not a gimmick here . . . it's just real food and real meals put together in an easy-to-use system. The true value, however, is that it is a plan you can live with long-term to maintain your weight. If you are despairing, as I was, that you could never get off the diet rollercoaster and 'just live a normal life,' please give *7 Systems Plan* a chance."

—Candy Boustead

Paperback: 978-1-64085-877-0
Hardback: 978-1-64085-878-7
Ebook: 978-1-64085-879-4

Library of Congress Control Number: 2019913002

The information included in this book is for educational purposes only. It does not replace any medical advice by your physician. The reader should regularly consult a physician in matters relating to health and particularly with respect to any symptoms that may require diagnosis or medical attention. It is highly recommended that you should always consult your medical physician before beginning any new diet, exercise, or health program. The information contained herein is provided without any representations or warranties, be they express or implied. Mention of specific companies, organizations, or authorities does not imply endorsement by the author or publisher, nor does mention of specific companies, organizations, or authorities imply that they endorse this book, its author, or publisher. The publisher and the author disclaim any liability for any medical outcomes that may occur as a result of the application of methods suggested in this book.

Some names and identifying details have been changed for confidentiality.

Dedication

To my wife, Teresa, my bright and shining morning star, whose inner and outer beauty have inspired and brought out the best in me.

Contents

Foreword

It's not often that I read a book and immediately change the way I think and act. However, after I read *7 Systems Plan*, everything changed—including what I ate for my next meal.

As Dr. Pat Luse eloquently proves, your body is a well-designed creation. Every System in it—if running correctly—should do its job. However, if one or more of your Systems is compromised, then your entire body could grind to a halt.

This reminds me of an unfortunate event that happened to me the other day in, of all places, a pharmacy drive-through. My vehicle was working fine as I made a right turn into the parking lot. I pulled up to the window and put my car in park.

My three kids waited patiently as I told the pharmacist my last name in order to pick up a prescription. Suddenly, the engine sputtered, and warning lights flashed all across the dashboard.

I felt a twinge of panic shoot through my arms and legs. The pharmacist retrieved the prescription from the back and handed it to me. That's when everything went dead. The vehicle shut off completely.

I forced a smile at the pharmacist and turned the key. Nothing. The engine didn't even turn over.

Besides feeling embarrassed for unintentionally becoming an obstruction, I was also confused. I knew the vehicle was in excellent condition, and it even had a new battery.

I had been cruising down the highway only an hour before, but in that moment, my car wasn't moving anywhere. It had ground to a halt.

After several unsuccessful attempts to "jump" the engine, I called in an expert—the local tow truck. A few minutes later, it removed my vehicle from the drive-through.

The next day, the service station identified the issue—a faulty alternator. Although the car was well maintained, one compromised part shut down the electrical system, which in turn sabotaged the entire vehicle. Several hundred dollars later, the mechanic fixed the alternator, which fixed the electrical system, and the engine roared back to life.

The story about my car and our bodies are related. One failing System will shut down everything else. Before we can start moving down the road of life again, we must repair our body's failing System. Sometimes, we need to bring in an expert to diagnose the issue. Dr. Pat Luse is that expert.

This book was designed to help you diagnose your compromised Systems. Once you get them working for you instead of against you, you'll experience amazing health transformations and lasting weight loss.

If you're ready to roar back to life, then you've picked the right book. Now all you need to do is buckle up for an exciting ride!

Kary Oberbrunner, author of *Elixir Project*,
Day Job to Dream Job, *The Deeper Path*,
and *Your Secret Name*

Acknowledgements

I would like to extend my sincere thanks to the following people:

My "team":

> My wife, Teresa, for her ideas, input, proofing, and patience during all the early mornings.
>
> My daughter-in-law Julie, for making the complexities simple and helping me find my voice.
>
> Kary Oberbrunner and his team at AAE, who have made this project a reality.

My many teachers and friends:

> Jonathan Wright, MD, whose stories in *Prevention Magazine* when I was a teenager gave me a vision for

someday using natural methods to help people with health problems.

Jeff Bland, PhD, for his relentless work scouring medical research and teaching me and countless others how to use this information to help patients regain their health.

NutriDyn, for the wealth of information they have supplied me over the last two decades in their seminars, as well as the world class supplements they produce for me and my patients.

The great team at my office who have helped me transform countless patients and refine the 7 Systems Plan.

My daughter-in-law Lori, for her insights and thoughts.

"Doc" Smith, my mentor and partner for many years.

Dr. Kurt Vollers, a fellow traveler on this journey in pursuit of health, science, and nutrition knowledge.

My mom, who owned and helped run a health food store until the age of 85.

The Functional Medicine Institute, that gave me the tools to turn science-based medicine into a practical treatment program.

The American Academy of Antiaging Medicine, for its ongoing cutting-edge, alternative medicine training.

My countless patients, whose life transformations after applying the principles you will learn in this book have inspired me to help even more people.

And finally, God, for His blessings and giving my life purpose.

Introduction

If you're like me, you're often tempted to skip the introduction. But doing so with this book could be hazardous to your health. Literally. You won't be able to have an amazing health transformation, lose weight, or heal chronic illness until you understand how to implement the 7 Systems Plan.

Here's the Cold Hard Truth

As of 2017, 76% of all Americans are overweight. At the current rate, 100% will be overweight by the year 2048.[1]

We've all been there. We go on a health kick, pick the latest diet plan, and start losing weight. Then something happens, we get off track, and get every pound back—plus some. Many studies reveal that 80% of people gain 90% of their weight back within one year.

This yo-yo dieting, or "weight cycling," can be very hard on your body. Every time you go on the typical diet, you lose muscle as well as fat. When you regain the weight, you don't get more muscle. You just take on extra fat. This phenomenon slows down your metabolism, making it even harder to keep weight off in the future.

A study of *The Biggest Loser*'s contestants showed that their metabolism had slowed by 700 calories during the competition and remained lower when they were done! On top of that, a year later, almost all of them had regained most of their weight.[2]

Diet and exercise alone rarely produce long-term weight loss. In Chapter One you'll meet one of my patients, Mary, who tried it for years. She went on countless diets, lost hundreds of pounds, and gained it all back. Following the 7 Systems Plan, she lost 105 pounds and has kept it off for the last 14 years.

Why It Is Not Your Fault

In an age of information overload—with thousands of diet and health programs available—we are more overweight and unhealthy than at any other time in our history. Almost all weight-loss programs fail to address the system malfunctions that cause weight gain. They fail because of these seven design flaws:

1. **Unhealthy Calorie Restriction:** You restrict calories in an unhealthy way, so your body defends itself by burning up to 300 fewer calories per day.
2. **Bad Bacteria:** You fail to address the bad bacteria in your gut that constantly send powerful signals to your brain to eat more junk food.
3. **Improper Food:** The food you choose may be "diet food," but it is not what your body needs, and that compromises the body's ability to burn fat.
4. **Useless Exercise:** The exercise program you choose is not efficient, so in spite of the time and effort you put into it, you burn few calories, make little progress, and fail to build muscle.

5. **Ineffective Communication**: Key hormones and brain neurotransmitters are not correctly balanced making you crave carbohydrates, be hungry, depressed, emotional and angry,

6. **Vulnerable Defense**: Because you are overweight, you have low-grade chronic inflammation. Besides not feeling well, you crave the wrong foods and gain more weight.

7. **Inefficient Detoxification:** Because your body's detoxification system is overwhelmed and compromised, your weight problems are compounded.

These seven design flaws take their toll on the majority of the population. The chance of an obese person (someone with a body mass index, or BMI, of 30) attaining normal body weight is 1 in 210 for men and 1 in 124 for women. These are not good odds. If you are severely obese (BMI of 40), these odds increase to 1 in 1,290 for men and 1 in 677 for women. Diet, exercise, and even willpower are not enough.

Despite these cold hard truths, there is hope. I've witnessed far too many transformations to think otherwise. Most people come to me completely discouraged and ready to give up. In a matter of days after beginning the 7 Systems Plan, they begin experiencing visible results. For the first time, they address the problem instead of just the pain.

A New Approach

While most diet plans (and traditional medical care) target the symptoms (the fruit), the 7 Systems Plan addresses the underlying malfunction that causes the symptoms (the root).

I have used the 7 Systems Plan to treat and transform the lives of countless overweight and ill patients. This model has evolved over the last two decades and includes the latest scientific breakthroughs to produce optimal results. In an effort to reach more people, I have now put the plan into this book and an online course.

The 7 Systems Plan can be summed up by the following points:

- Your body is a network of seven key Systems (Structural, Digestive, Delivery, Energy, Communication, Defense, Detox).
- These Systems are interdependent and affect each other.
- The correct function of each System has a significant impact on your overall health and weight.
- Patients should be treated individually, based on their specific System needs.
- There are simple steps to help each System function optimally.

The 7 Systems Plan is a new lifestyle that comes from a new way of thinking: Most weight problems and diseases occur when one or more of your Systems are not functioning properly.

In this book, our strategy is threefold. We'll evaluate your Systems, identify the imbalances or malfunctions, and then optimize your Systems.

The 7 System Strategy

Evaluate —> Identify —> Optimize

It might sound like work until you remember the benefits: amazing health transformations and lasting weight loss. If you are ready to experience these benefits, then keep reading.

The Solution: The 7 Systems Plan

Your body is an incredible network of Systems. If all of your Systems are working well, you'll have an ideal weight and optimal health. In today's world—because of our toxic environment, processed food, and stress-driven lifestyle—it is not easy for each System to function optimally. If one System sputters, your weight goes up and your health goes down. In a matter of days, a domino effect can take down your other Systems.

The key to permanent weight loss and optimal health is to fix all seven of these Systems.

Running the human body efficiently and effectively requires all of the Systems to work together in alignment. This renovation process begins with correcting the *Structural System* (bone, muscle, and fat). This System houses all of your body's other Systems.

Your *Digestive System* takes food in and breaks it down into a form that can enter the bloodstream. Your brain is intricately wired to this System. Mastering this component also masters your waistline.

The *Delivery System* picks up the nutrients from the Digestive System and transports them through the bloodstream into the cells where they can be used. Healthy eating does not help if nutrients can't get into the cells. The 7 Systems Plan gets the right food delivered to the cells for maximum weight loss.

After nutrients enter the cell, they are converted into fuel by the *Energy System*. In the upcoming chapters, you'll discover how to get up to 600% more energy in a short amount of time. Imagine what you could do with 600% more energy!

Your *Communication System* enables all of the Systems to "talk" with one another, ensuring proper function. You'll experience faster weight loss and fewer cravings when your hormones, nerves, and neurotransmitters can communicate.

Your body is exposed to harmful substances every day, and you need an adequate *Defense System* to protect you from them. Fixing this System will reduce chronic inflammation, making it much easier to lose weight fast and stay healthy.

And lastly, your body's *Detox System* cleans up after all of this work has been done. Toxins make you fat, and the 7 Systems Plan minimizes toxins.

The Results

The 7 Systems Plan will help you get to your ideal weight fast and keep the pounds off for good. But weight loss is not the only benefit. You'll also reduce your risk of death from all causes by a whopping 80%!

Many of my patients have eliminated their diabetes, unclogged heart arteries, corrected hormone imbalances, overcome depression, cleared up chronic skin problems, reduced or eliminated their medications, and much more by following this plan. Men and women declare that they feel years younger.

After following the 7 Systems Plan for a short time, your cravings and appetite will decrease significantly while your mental function and mood improve. The best part is that after you understand how your Systems work and implement this plan, your results are likely to be permanent. The more aware you become, the better equipped you are to make healthier choices for the rest of your life.

When your Systems are all functioning as they should, you'll maintain an ideal weight, optimize your overall health, experience higher energy levels, and live a longer, disease-free life.

By the way, if you're looking for a doctor who tells you to eat only organic vegetables, never have junk food, and eat brussels sprouts every day, then I am not your doctor. You can have a little fun and still be healthy!

In the next seven chapters, we'll unpack each of the seven Systems one at a time for maximum understanding. We'll use these four questions as our framework:

1. **What?** A brief introduction to the System.
2. **Who?** Meet a patient whose System was working against them.
3. **Why?** A look at why this System is working against you.
4. **How?** Proven steps to get this System working for you.

Your body is a well-designed creation. Every System plays a vital role in your overall wellness. Our goal is simple: get these Systems to function correctly so you can have amazing health transformations, lose weight, and heal chronic illness. If you are ready, let's get started on your path to weight loss, health, and vitality!

—Dr. Pat Luse

1

The Structural System
Bone, Muscle, and Fat

Don't let your angry fat keep killing you.

Startling Facts:

- It is estimated that half of all Americans over the age of 50 are at risk for bone problems. Worldwide, loss of bone density causes an osteoporotic fracture every three seconds.[3]
- Without intervention, you can lose seven pounds of muscle per decade. Muscle loss with aging (sarcopenia) is the most important indicator of health as you get older.[4]
- The more you overstuff your fat cells, the more they will sabotage your health. One in five U.S. deaths is related to obesity.[5]

"Get the *structure* right, and the *function* will follow!"
—Linus Pauling

A Brief Introduction to The Structural System

The Structural System is the foundation for all the other Systems because it holds everything together. Your bones, muscles, and fat perform these three vital functions:

1. Bone = Supports
2. Muscle = Moves
3. Fat = Stores

Let's unpack each of these functions one at a time.

Bone: The Support Function

Many times, we don't value this System until it's out of alignment. If you've ever suffered from joint pain, stiffness, broken bones, or a misaligned spine, you probably have an appreciation for a properly functioning Structural System.

Our bones, cartilage, and tissues support our bodies. Strong bones are necessary because they protect our brain, spinal cord, and vital organs. Our bones store important minerals and house white blood cells, which are essential for immune function.

Unfortunately, many people have discovered how unhealthy bones can eliminate their independence, invite disease, and cause death. Loss of bone health can affect your spine, arms, and legs. 24% of people with a hip fracture die within the next year.[6] The consequences of neglecting your bones will also affect your mobility and independence. After suffering a hip fracture, 40% of people are unable to walk independently, 60% require assistance a year later, and 33% are totally dependent or in a nursing home the following year.[7]

Muscle: The Move Function

Without muscles, we couldn't move. Thankfully, we have about 700 muscles attached to our bones. Skeletal muscle mass is comprised of muscle tissue, blood vessels, nerves, and tendons, and it should make up about 30–50% of your body weight.

Muscles enable us to walk, talk, eat, sit, and stand, but they also assist in small movements like facial expressions and breathing. We need voluntary muscles (those we consciously control, like arms and legs) and involuntary muscles (those we don't consciously control, like our heart and intestinal tract).

As with our bones, we might take our muscles for granted. However, they're a critical component of wellness. As your muscle mass decreases, you lose strength and mobility and your metabolism slows down. Studies show that muscle mass is the most important factor in predicting health as we get older.

The good news is that this loss is not inevitable. You can regain muscle mass with the 7 Systems Plan.

Fat: The Storage Function

Protein, fat, and carbohydrates provide your body with essential fuel. If these nutrients are not used right away, they go into storage. Your liver and muscles can store about 1,500 calories of carbohydrate as glucose. Compare this to the 40,000 (or more) calories stored as fat in the fat cells.

Fat isn't necessarily a bad thing. We need to have energy reserves for times of need. But while these reserves are important, we live in a society where times of need are few and far between. As a result, excess calories continue to increase our fat reserve.

To make matters worse, most of us have genes that allow our bodies to store this energy far too efficiently! Geneticists are calling it the "thrifty" gene. While some people seem able to eat whatever they want and not gain a pound, the majority of us never enjoy this experience. Instead, our bodies are good at taking the extra calories and storing them on our bellies!

7 Signs That Your Structural System Is Working Against You:

1. Weight gain (particularly fat stored around the belly)
2. Osteoporosis or osteopenia
3. Back and neck pain
4. Loss of height
5. Loss of strength and decreased muscle tone
6. Waist measurement larger than your hips
7. Weak memory or mental fog

Meet Mary

One afternoon, I gave a lecture in my office to a room full of men and women who had a desire to experience better health. When I'd finished my presentation, I closed my laptop and began gathering my notes. From the corner of my eye, I saw a woman with poor posture and a slight limp walking toward me. When she spoke, I immediately picked up a twinge of panic in her voice. "I am 60 years old and about to retire from my job. It hurts too much to work. What hurts even more is that I won't be here for my grandkids if I don't do something fast."

Sensing the urgency of her situation, I set up an evaluation right away. I wanted to identify the cause of her poor health and severe weight problems.

In her consultation, she told me she had been on countless diets and lost hundreds of pounds, only to gain them all back and more. She had given up hope of having her thin body back. She also had joint problems, and she'd recently had a knee replaced.

Examination and lab testing revealed that she suffered from hypertension, high cholesterol, inflammation, and type 2 diabetes. A body composition evaluation showed severe muscle loss and over 100 pounds of extra body fat. Her skeletal exam revealed osteopenia, a forward head posture, an increased curve in the thoracic spine, and degenerative joint disease. She was already on prescription drugs and would be placed on more if she pursued medical treatment for her conditions. Based on her history, the examination, and lab tests, I decided to focus on her Structural System.

Over the course of the next year, Mary followed the 7 Systems Plan and eliminated her need for prescription medicine. Her blood pressure and cholesterol normalized, and her type 2 diabetes disappeared. She gained significant muscle and lost over 100 pounds of body fat. Spinal adjustments improved her posture and bone and joint health tremendously. In addition to feeling great, she looked so different that many people did not recognize her.

The key to her success was fixing her malfunctioning Structural System and then optimizing the other Systems. Once we did that, we eliminated most of her health problems. This truth proves an important point that we'll revisit throughout the book: When the body's Systems are all functioning correctly, weight loss and health are a normal result.

Even 14 years after our initial assessment, Mary has kept the weight off and maintained a healthy Structural System by following the 7 Systems Plan.

Why Your Bones Are Working Against You

Lifestyle choices such as smoking, drinking, poor diet, and consuming soft drinks are known to interfere with the body's ability to absorb calcium. These behaviors slow down new bone formation. Some medications are known to adversely affect the health and building of bones, especially statin (cholesterol-lowering) drugs, antidepressants, and proton pump inhibitors (acid reflux drugs). Hormone deficiencies can also impair bone building. See Chapter Five for more hormone information.

Your body is comprised of 206 different bones, and the alignment of these bones is critical. At one time or another, you may have "thrown your back out" or been unable to turn your neck. These injuries indicate deeper structural problems that—if left untreated—can have serious consequences. Altered structure causes altered function.

This phenomenon is often seen in the spine. Misalignments in the spine can affect nerve function, and that in turn can affect organ function. More and more studies reveal that spinal manipulation not only helps maintain correct spinal alignment, joint mobility, and disc health, but it can also affect proper nerve function.[8]

Spinal issues are the number one reason that people aged 50 and older are forced to quit working, but these issues are quickly becoming more common for the younger generation. I'm alarmed by the number of young people who come to me with degenerative disc and degenerative joint disease in the spine. Lifestyle, trauma, and unaddressed alignment problems contribute to this degeneration.

How to Get Your Bones Working for You

1. Add bone-building nutrients to your diet:
   - Calcium: greens, seeds, and beans
   - Magnesium: nuts and seeds
   - Vitamin K1: green vegetables
2. Eat lean meat and plant protein: beans, seeds, and nuts.
3. Take bone-healthy supplements: Vitamin D3 and Vitamin K2.
4. Avoid foods that cause calcium loss: excess sodium, soft drinks, and caffeine.
5. Do weight-bearing exercises: weight training, walking, jogging, etc.
6. Keep your pH neutral (more on this in Chapter Six).
7. Fix your hormones.

Why Your Muscles Are Working Against You

If you don't use it, you lose it—and most people have. If you do not eat the foods your body needs and exercise, you lose your flexibility and strength as you age. Tendons shorten, joints become stiff, muscles waste away, and your energy goes down. Because you have less muscle, your metabolism slows. It becomes harder to lose weight, so fat increases.

Loss of muscle mass can also lead to an overall decline in metabolic and hormone function. Ignoring muscle loss leads to reduced strength, accelerated aging, and increased risk of chronic illnesses like diabetes and heart disease.

How to Get Your Muscles Working for You

How you move determines the amount of muscle you have and the speed at which your body ages. Choosing when you eat is just as important as what you eat. By consuming healthy calories at the appropriate levels at the right times, you'll increase hormone production that will, in turn, build and maintain muscle mass.

Chapter Four (The Energy System) will give you the secrets to the fast muscle-gain program that helped Mary go from deconditioned to fit in a short time.

Why Your Fat Is Working Against You

The most common defect in the Structural System is with the storage function, specifically the way your body stores fat. If you stuff a fat cell too much, it quickly becomes your enemy instead of your ally. We call these "angry" fat cells.

When you take in nutrients but do not use them right away, they eventually end up in fat cells. We used to think of these fat cells as silent, ugly cells that just sit there. Now we know that they can swell up to six times their normal size and send "distress" signal molecules (called adipokines) throughout your body.

The adipokines trigger the production of various chemicals and hormones that make you eat more, burn fewer calories, have higher blood pressure, experience inflammation, and even get cancer.

The more you overstuff your fat cells, the more they will sabotage your health. Think of them as selfish, angry children who suck up all the calories in your bloodstream, behave badly, and make life miserable for everyone.

Of all the places that you store fat, the belly is the most dangerous. When fat begins to accumulate here, it also builds up in your organs, affecting your heart, brain, liver, kidneys, and pancreas. Angry fat cells negatively affect these organs and can even cause them to die.

To lose weight and feel better, you must target these angry fat cells. This is an important fix so we will spend a lot of time on it.

All seven of your Systems can make these fat cells angry. But first, let's talk about your genes' role in this problem.

It's tempting to blame genes as the cause of weight gain and fat storage problems. But there's a problem with that. Although heredity is an important factor, it turns out that we have more control than was once thought possible.

You are not your genes—or at least, you don't have to be. Years ago, we assumed that if you had good genes, you'd "made" it. You'd be healthy and live a long life.

We now know that genes only play a small role in determining our weight, health, and longevity. According to Dan Buettner, author of *Blue Zone*, genetics is only 10% of the story while lifestyle is the other 90%. This theory is confirmed by studies that reveal that 80–90% of all cancer and most diseases are caused by what you do to your genes.[9]

Here is why genes are not as important a factor as we once thought: Bad genes can either be turned on or silenced. Many of us carry genes that make us more susceptible to obesity, cancer, diabetes, and many other health problems. Every time you eat, the food sends information to these genes. A poor diet can activate bad genes and turn off good ones.

The 7 Systems Plan empowers you to change all of this. Each time you take a bite of food, you're sending signals to your genes. It has been shown that about three months after moving to a healthy lifestyle, men had changes in activity in 501 genes. 48 genes were turned on, and 453 were turned off.

That sounds amazing—and it is. In the remaining chapters, you'll discover how to turn off your own bad genes and turn on the genes that make you lose weight, look younger, and feel younger!

How to Get Your Fat Working for You

Step 1: Inventory your intake.

Before we can begin to fix this System, we need to examine what is going into your body. A person of average weight underestimates what they consume by 20%. Overweight people underestimate what they consume by 30–50%.

To fully understand what you consume and how much you consume, you must keep track and write it down. Thanks to technology, it's not as much work as it sounds. Besides, the benefits make this a worthy investment of your time. All of my patients have told me that this is research they don't regret.

In this first step, don't adjust what you eat or how much you eat. Just accurately record everything. It may surprise you. The typical American male consumes 3,770 calories per day—and 1/3 of that is junk food. Journaling is one of the most powerful ways to regain control of your eating. My patients have doubled their weight loss by implementing this one step.

What you need:

- A journal
- A calorie nutrition book
- Three different colored pens, markers, or highlighters (green, yellow, and red)

What you do:

- Record the date and time
- Write down exactly what you eat and drink, including water and other beverages.
- Refer to the food journal in Part Three of Appendix A: Resources.

If you prefer an app or website to keep track of what you consume, my patients have found the following tools extremely helpful:

- My Fitness Pal
- Fit Day
- My Calorie Counter

You can access these at 7SystemsPlan.com. If you choose the digital app route, you will be able to see your weekly summary and nutrient-weak areas and track your success.

1. **Identify your Food.**

Categorize the real foods you eat and those that aren't considered real foods. All the food you eat will fall into one of three categories: real, processed, and ultra-processed.

In America, less than 1% of calories come from vegetables. About 30% of calories come from minimally processed foods, and a whopping 57% of calories come from ultra-processed foods.[10]

At the end of a week, use different colors to identify the categories of food you ate.

Real Food: *Green means go*. Anything that is directly from the vine, bush, tree, or earth is considered real food. This includes foods that are unprocessed or minimally processed:

- Fresh or frozen fruits and vegetables
- Nuts and seeds
- Legumes (beans)
- Eggs
- 100% whole grains
- Lean meats
- Foods that contain no added sugar

Only about one in five people get more than 75% of their calories from real food. This should be the biggest part of your diet.

Processed Foods: *Yellow means use caution.* This category includes some bread, pasta, most canned foods, oils, cheese, some meat, most dairy, and often things in a bag or box. Processing food frequently involves the depletion of nutrients and the addition of ingredients that may not be healthy. Some foods in this category are acceptable while others are not.

You can eat some processed food, but choose wisely. Here are some acceptable items:

- Sugar-free applesauce
- Canned and dried beans
- Guacamole
- Hummus
- Real avocado oil mayonnaise
- Olives
- Organic broth
- Peanut butter (refrigerated with no hydrogenated oils or sugar)
- Low-sugar pickles
- Pumpkin (not pie filling)
- Tomato sauces (glass jars with no sugar added)
- Canned or frozen wild-caught salmon, mackerel, and sardines
- Unsweetened yogurt

Ultra-Processed Foods: *Red means stop.* Items that fit into this category have been significantly altered from their source. These foods contain excessive amounts of sugar and bad fats as well as many chemical additives. These ultra-processed foods are the worst of the worst, and you should strictly limit your intake:

- Most breads
- Breakfast cereals
- Chips
- Soft drinks
- Refined grains
- Pizza
- Frozen pre-made meals
- Sauces
- Instant soups and foods

2. **Calculate your Calories.**

Calculate the total calories that you consume each day. Make sure you're accurate about the portion size and calories for everything on your list. When you're done, total the calories at the end of each day.

If you want to know how much real food you are eating, add up the calories from each of the three categories (green, yellow, red) and figure out the percentage of your total diet coming from each category.

I've included free printable journaling pages as well as many other tools at 7SystemsPlan.com.

3. **Review your Journal.**

Look at your journal and see how much red and yellow there is. How do you feel about your results? Don't judge yourself. Remember, awareness is always the first step of any breakthrough. Most people will realize that one-third of their diet comes from junk food (ultra-processed food).

Read Labels

Losing weight means being aware of what you consume. Read the nutrition facts on everything you eat, and pay special attention to these elements:
- Serving Size: There may be more than one serving in the package. A bag of potato chips might say it has 150 calories per serving, but the entire bag might contain three servings (450 calories).
- Calories: Total calories in one serving.
- Protein, Fat, and Carbohydrate: Avoid all forms of sugar, hydrogenated oils, and trans fats.
- Fiber: The more, the better.
- Ingredients: The product's ingredients are listed in order of quantity, so those with the largest amounts come first.

Step 2: Educate and eliminate.

If you knew that a particular kind of fuel was destroying your vehicle, you wouldn't keep putting it in the tank. The same goes for your body—some foods will destroy it, and some will increase performance. Even if something tastes good, it could be destroying you.

In Step 1, you inventoried your intake. This new education made you aware of the "red" and "yellow" categories of food that are hurting you.

In this step, you have the opportunity to act on this education and begin eliminating overstuffed fat cells. Remember, overstuffed cells turn into angry fat cells. You might wonder why it's so important to fix your diet. According to the most rigorous analysis of risk factors ever published, the number one cause of death and disability in the United States is a poor diet.[11] Eating real food in proper amounts will silence angry fat cells, increase your lifespan, and decrease disease.

The key is to eat more real food and get the right amounts of protein, fat, and carbohydrates. These two actions eliminate 80% of the barriers to maintaining proper weight and health!

Besides avoiding the ultra-processed food, you'll also need to be intentional about how much food you ingest because excess carbohydrates and proteins will convert to glucose and get stored as fat.

Balancing the quantities of fat, protein, and carbohydrates that you take in will also give you more energy. Starving yourself is counterproductive. It throws your body into fat-conservation mode. When this happens, your metabolism slows down and you burn less fat.

Step 3: Implement the 7 Systems Plan.

After decades of study, clinical practice, and working with count-less patients, I have crafted a unique plan to help you lose weight and fix your Systems. I've synthesized the best of the best in scientific research and my decades of experience to create the 7 Systems Plan.

Throughout the remainder of this book, we'll unpack the 7 Systems Plan in its entirety. For now, let's take a look at what foods will benefit your Structural System.

Everybody would benefit from eating more vegetables and good fats. Don't just take my word for it!

You may remember the story of Daniel in the Bible. Daniel asks permission to remain on a vegetable and water diet instead of eating the king's choice foods and wine (probably something like the average American diet). After 10 days on this plan, Daniel and his friends were found to be smarter and better looking than those who ate the king's diet.

I have no doubt that God influenced the results of this test, but I also know that God

7 Benefits of The 7 Systems Plan

1. Helps You Lose Weight
2. Improves Heart Health
3. Helps Fight Cancer
4. Prevents and Treats Diabetes
5. Protects Cognitive Health
6. Prolongs Life
7. Helps You De-Stress and Relax

can use natural things to accomplish his plan. A recent study from Saint Andrews University concluded that people who ate three additional daily portions of produce for six weeks were ranked as better looking than those who didn't.[12] Another recent study shows that vegetables help you feel calmer, improve your mental well-being, and may increase your curiosity and creativity.[13]

Vegetables are known to improve good health and function, athletic performance, energy, and mood. They also boost immune function and decrease cancer risk. Because different colors of vegetables contain different nutrients, it is important to "eat the rainbow." Cruciferous vegetables are some of the most important (these include broccoli, cauliflower, and cabbage).

You should also eat more fat. However, it needs to be the right kind of fat.

Consider the facts of this eye-opening study. People were assigned to one of three groups that were followed for over four years:

- Group A: Mediterranean diet supplemented with one liter of extra virgin olive oil per week
- Group B: Mediterranean diet supplemented with 30 grams of nuts per day
- Group C: Low-fat diet

Guess who won for brain function, heart disease, and stroke?

Brain Results:

- Group A: Olive oil group experienced significantly improved cognition.
- Group B: Nuts group showed significant improvement in memory.
- Group C: Low-fat group showed a significant *decrease* in both memory and cognitive function.

Heart and Stroke Risk Results:

- Group A: Olive oil group showed a 49% stroke reduction.
- Group B: Nuts group showed a 30% relative risk reduction for cardiovascular disease.
- Group C: Low-fat group had to be stopped for ethical reasons.

Clearly, the low-fat group lost.[14]

Foods to Eat

In Appendix A, Part One, I give a complete shopping list of beneficial foods, but here is a quick overview:

*Foods you should eat a **lot more** of:*

- Consume at least 5–10 cups per day of low-sugar vegetables. In the shopping list, I give you 50 to choose from. This should cover at least half of your plate at each meal.

  Note: I've seen patients who had never eaten vegetables before succeed on this plan. One man had not eaten a vegetable (other than potatoes) for 20 years! At 7SystemsPlan. com, you'll discover many ways to eat more vegetables. You can stir fry, bake, puree, or juice them to make them enjoyable. I also include a printable shopping list so that you can stock your kitchen with real food.

*Foods you should eat **some** of:*

- Foods high in healthy fat (avocados, nuts, olives, seeds)
- Healthy meats (ideally grass fed, antibiotic free, and hormone free)
- Fish (wild caught, low mercury, and high in omega-3 fatty acid)
- Eggs (ideally organic, high in omega-3, free-range)
- Low-sugar fruits (apples, berries, oranges, pears, etc.)

- Functional foods for ultra-fast progress (discussed more in Chapter Three)

*Foods you should eat a **little** of:*

- Extra virgin olive oil, coconut oil, real mayonnaise with avocado oil
- Legumes (beans, split peas, lentils), though limit these if you have inflammation and blood sugar problems. Although they are good for you, they contain lectins which can be proinflammatory. To remove these toxins, always soak beans in water for at least 12 hours before cooking them at least 15 minutes on high heat.
- Medium-sugar vegetables (carrots, sweet potatoes, winter squash, beets, Yukon Gold potatoes, pumpkins)
- High-sugar fruits (bananas, pineapples, dried fruits)
- Whole grains (quinoa, brown rice, rolled oats), try to avoid gluten
- Nuts and seeds

*Foods you should use **sparingly**:*

- Sweeteners (sugar, maple syrup, honey, stevia, and xylitol)
- Cultured dairy (cheese and butter/ghee, yogurt—ideally plain or homemade)

*Foods you should **avoid** altogether:*

- Milk (substitute almond, hemp, and coconut milk—no sugar added)
- High-sugar vegetables (potatoes)
- Most processed and all ultra-processed foods
- Artificial sweeteners and food additives

Remember, the 7 Systems Plan is about making your Systems work for you, not against you. You will probably increase your food volume because real food takes up a large amount of space despite having fewer calories.

Does this mean no more junk food ever? While that is the ideal, few can do it. So, if you need to, have a little. If you lose control when you eat junk food, completely avoid it. Some people must draw a hard line between foods they can and can't have. Foods containing sugar, white flour, and bad fats tend to cause the greatest addiction and loss of self-control. Keeping these out of your diet is a key to your success.

Although I want you to watch calories, I don't believe that eating well is only about calories. If you're limiting calories or portion size but eating the wrong food, you'll probably be hungry and feel deprived. This creates a brand-new set of problems.

Sustainable success comes from having each of your Systems working optimally. By choosing quality calories (nutrient-dense food that is also real), you'll feel full and happy and be able to provide the necessary fuel your body needs to perform at its full potential.

Eventually, you won't need to be concerned about calories at all. Your Systems will work correctly, and you'll be proficient at eating nutrient-dense foods that taste appealing too. But in the beginning, you must become aware of the calories that you consume because your misconceptions about the quality and quantity of your food are possibly what got you where you are in the first place.

Don't worry. I make eating better simple with the tools and resources in Appendix A. My plan will show you how to consume quality calories. At first, it takes some work, but as you read each chapter and learn, it gets easier and easier. In Chapter Three, we'll talk about macronutrients and micronutrients. For now, we'll keep things as simple as possible: You must learn to distinguish real food from its imposter.

Dr. Pat's 95% Rule

You only have to eat healthy 95% of the time to be very healthy and get an A+ on the 7 Systems Plan.

Step 4: Change your fuel sources.

Dr. Ron Rosedale said, "Your health, and likely your lifespan, will be determined by the proportion of fat versus sugar you burn in your lifetime." There are few things in life as powerful as being a good "fat burner."

Unfortunately, many people have lost the ability to burn fat for fuel. Instead, fat becomes locked up in their bodies and cannot be used as energy. The 7 Systems Plan reverses this.

Here's how.

Your body has two fuels it can utilize: stored fat or calories from your diet. You might wonder why your body can't use stored fat as energy instead of storing additional fat in unwanted places. The answer is simple—your body prefers to run off of dietary carbohydrates (glucose). The more overweight you are, the harder it is to run on anything but carbohydrates. It is the default fuel your body uses when plenty of calories and carbohydrates are coming in.

Eating too many calories or bad carbohydrates leads to fat storage, weight gain, and the inability to burn fat for fuel. But when reserves of glucose (glycogen) are depleted, your body is forced to burn stored fat for fuel. Most people have weeks or even months of energy stored as fat. Going longer periods of time between eating or eating less than your body needs, as recommended by the 7 Systems Plan, can force your body to become better at burning stored fat.

When my patients first start this program, the only time they get close to burning fat is in the morning, after they've gone all night without eating. Most people aren't used to letting their bodies run out of their first choice for fuel (glucose), so their bodies aren't good at using stored fat. However, in time, your body will eventually catch on. Plus, there are ways to make this easier. The more you use your fat for fuel, the better your body gets at releasing fat when needed.

Fixing the Structural System will up-regulate the enzymes and hormones necessary to make your body a proficient fat burner. You'll get to the point where your body can easily release stored fat when it needs energy. As a result, you'll have less hunger and plenty of energy. This component is critical if you want to feel better and slow down the aging process.

When you use stored fat for energy, it starts a domino effect. For starters, your body loves this fuel source, and your weight will decrease. But in addition to that, the 7 Systems Plan reverses chronic and debilitating illnesses. Many of my patients no longer need prescription drugs. Instead, they testify to looking and feeling 5–10 years younger than they did when they began the program.

The 7 Systems Plan works whether or not you restrict calories. As a result, you might wonder why you should bother reducing your calories. The rationale is simple: this tweak is one of the most powerful steps you can take to achieve your health goals faster. It shifts your progress into overdrive.

That's why the rest of this chapter is dedicated to showing you how to restrict calories properly. We want to make your body a great fat burner. The first week or two may seem difficult, but soon you'll have more energy. You'll wake up happier and feel better about yourself and your efforts toward weight loss and optimal health.

The 7 Systems Plan tells your genes what to do and prevents angry fat cells from communicating with the rest of your body.

Defining Calories

Calories are essential for all living things. They're the energy currency your body needs. There's a tremendous difference between the various types of calories and the effect they have on you. Not all calories are created equal:

- Some cause damage while others heal.
- Some speed up your metabolism while others slow it down.
- Some decrease your appetite while others increase it.
- Some fill you up while others leave you wanting more.

Although calories are essential for life, consuming more than enough overfills your cells, causing your Systems to function improperly. In this scenario, too much of a good thing is definitely a bad thing. And in the American diet, it's obvious that calories have become a bad thing for the majority of people. Today we are consuming 500 more calories per day than we did in 1970.

> A candy bar and five apples have the same number of calories, but their effects on your hormones and Systems are drastically different. One will make you gain weight and do damage, and the other will make you lose weight and repair.

Deleting Calories

The thought of restricting calories conjures up all sorts of uncomfortable imagery —going without your favorite foods for the rest of your life or worrying about never eating out with friends again. But it does not have to be this way. You can enjoy food while still restricting calories.

Calorie restriction, when done properly, has the following effects:

- Slows down and reverses the aging process
- Makes you significantly healthier and stronger
- Protects you from toxins and stress
- Reduces free radical damage
- Decreases damage to your DNA, preventing 84 major gene changes
- Blocks the genes that cause cells to grow old
- Has been used to treat and prevent cancer
- Gives you more energy

Is it too late for you?

In one study, animals that started eating a restricted-calorie diet at middle age realized about 90% of the same benefits as animals that had been restricting calories since infancy. It's not too late!

Some experts have theorized that if you consumed 900 calories per day, you could live 200 years. This is hardly practical. If you did, you'd be hungry for 200 years. However, if you reduced your calorie intake by one-third, you could add 24 years to your life. Is this practical? Absolutely.

The truth is that reducing calories is the most powerful thing you can do for your body. This has been researched and proven time and time again. It's the most effective and efficient method to lose weight and get healthy.

The problem is that if it's the only thing you do, you're doomed to fail. Need proof? Take a peek at the millions of people who restrict calories and lose weight each year. What happens shortly thereafter? Most people gain it all back. For permanent results, we need to fix our Systems. Thankfully, the remainder of this book will show you how.

My diet is typically 1,000 calories less than the average American male. Don't be fooled though. If you examine the quantity of food I consume, it might be even more than the average American. It's not a matter of *how much*, but rather *what kind*. The food I choose is high in nutrients and volume but low in calories.

I'm a big fan of healthy *and* tasty. I can eat a 500-calorie meal that tastes wonderful and is so big that I can't even finish everything on my plate.

How to Restrict Calories And Not Be Hungry

Have you tried to restrict calories before? Nearly all diet plans integrate calorie restriction in some way. The chances are that you're using this strategy right now. Most people restrict calories improperly and feel perpetually hungry because of it.

You won't be hungry following the 7 Systems Plan because real food fills you up. At the same time, your Systems will start functioning as they should. Every week, I hear my patients say, "I am so full on your plan, and I feel so much better."

Trust me when I say that I've seen calorie restriction—done right—transform people's lives. By committing to this step, you will begin to experience benefits far beyond weight loss.

The idea is to eat in a way that satisfies you, making you feel better physically and mentally, while fixing your Systems. Losing weight is a desirable side benefit.

How many calories do you need per day?

Many people wonder how many calories they truly need. In Appendix A, Part Two, I offer a method to help you evaluate this number if you want to be exact. Generally, to keep your weight the same, the average female needs about 2,000 calories per day and the average male needs about 2,500 calories. You must go below this number or change the quality of those calories to lose weight. You should do both for maximum results.

I have my patients decrease their calorie intake by about 30%. So, if you have an average-sized body frame and you're a female, this means starting at 1,300 calories. If you're a male, this means starting at 1,600–1,900 calories. If you have a big frame, a very active job, or if you exercise frequently, you'll need more calories. I provide more details in Appendix A, Part Two.

If you restrict calories too much or eat the wrong calories, your metabolism will slow down and stay there. Combat this tendency by sticking with the foods I suggest and staying within the proper calorie range. My patients achieve the best short- and long-term results when they don't restrict calories the same amount every day. We'll discuss this in a minute.

By following the 7 Systems Plan, you'll convert to burning fat for energy. Notice the Calorie Equation©:

Quality Calories + Calorie Restriction = Maximum Results

$$(QC + CR = MR)$$

Give it some time, and it will get easier. Most people eat food continuously during the day, especially carbohydrates. As a result, your body downregulates the enzymes and hormones needed to burn up your fat reserves, making it harder for your body to get rid of stored fat. When you continually consume food, your body is always in building mode—building more fat on your body.

In the ideal world, your body works in two shifts.

First Shift: This is the nutrient intake phase. Proper food and vitamins are taken in, and these nutrients build a healthier body.

Second Shift: This is the fasting phase. When food is absent, your body switches into a different mode where it eliminates fat, repairs, and then rejuvenates. This is when your body does its necessary "house cleaning": removing garbage, repairing old cells, regenerating new cells, and eliminating malformed or cancerous cells. This is when your body uses stored fat for energy.

Many people never experience this second shift because they are constantly eating. As a result, they never experience these essential benefits either. Thankfully, there is a solution.

Discover Fasting

Fasting is an amazing practice, though it's hardly a new concept. Thousands of books have been written about its health benefits. Fasting will

- Prolong your life
- Normalize insulin and increase insulin sensitivity
- Decrease disease markers
- Normalize ghrelin (the hunger hormone)
- Repair, and regenerate tissues
- Increase human growth hormone (the youth hormone)
- Lower triglycerides
- Reduce inflammation and free radical damage
- Reduce markers of aging, diabetes, inflammation, heart disease, and cancer

In some circles, fasting has gotten a bad rap. Evidently, some people have equated it to starving. Myths about fasting reducing muscle mass or slowing down metabolism haven't helped either. These beliefs couldn't be farther from the truth. Fasting *maintains* muscle mass remarkably well and can even help "reset" your metabolism at a higher level.

Water-only fasting has many benefits, but if you have ever done it, you'll know that during the first two days you can feel hungry. Some of these feelings are caused by thinking about food, but hang in there; the hunger hormone is reduced over time and significantly decreases after two days.

Step 5: Experiment with "Fast-Mimicking Diets" (FMDs).

In my decades of helping patients get healthy, I have found that fasting can increase short- and long-term success by up to 80%. Now imagine having all the benefits of fasting while still being able to eat. New fasting techniques are called fast-mimicking diets (FMDs for short). These diets "trick" the brain into thinking that you are fasting although you haven't completely stopped eating food. "Intermittent fasting" and "time-restricted eating" are other terms for methods that restrict the time or amount we eat as a way of giving the body some time off from digestion to burn fat and repair.

The National Institute on Aging has presented its data on the benefits of fast-mimicking diets to the FDA. Once they receive approval, doctors can begin prescribing this kind of diet to treat and prevent diseases in their patients.

The primary researcher behind the studies, Valter Longo, says that the diet is a way to help the body reboot itself. "It's about reprograming the body so it enters a slower aging mode, but also rejuvenating it through stem cell-based regeneration and rejuvenation in multiple systems."[15]

One of the most exciting discoveries is that FMDs dramatically increase production of human growth hormone (HGH). This hormone is made by the pituitary gland (the master gland) and plays a huge role in the normal development of children and adolescents. However, it also plays a role in adults. If your HGH is low, it leads to higher levels of body fat (obesity), less muscle (sarcopenia), and decreased bone mass (osteopenia). Naturally, we want more HGH, but a surefire way to turn it off is to eat all the time.

Decades of studies have shown that an increase in HGH decreases fat mass and nearly doubles lean muscle mass. It also improves the skin's thickness over time. The bad news is that the synthetic version of the hormone has adverse side effects. The good news is that scientists and many professional athletes have discovered a strategy for secreting the hormone in an all-natural way: fasting. After rigorous testing, it's been found that fasting provides a 300% increase in this anti-aging hormone![15]

Although there are many versions of FMDs, I've included three of my favorites here. These are versions that both my patients and I use regularly:

- *The 17-Hour Fast*: Restrict your eating to a 7-hour window each day followed by a 17-hour fast. This method can be used daily.
- *The 23-Hour Fast*: Eat your evening meal and then fast until the next day's evening meal. This method can be used one to three times per week.
- *The 5:2 Fast*: Significantly restrict your calorie consumption two nonconsecutive days per week, consuming your regular number of calories on the other five days. This method can be used weekly.

I have personally used each of these plans for years, and I am amazed at the results: less hunger, more energy, greater weight loss, and effortless weight maintenance. I will expand on these three FMDs soon, but for now, you can start following the steps I've outlined below.

Month One: Get in a rhythm.
A simple plan is laid out in Appendix A, Parts One, Two and Three, but here is an overview:

- Read the tips to make the 7 Systems Plan work for you.
- Use the 7 Systems Plan shopping list to stock up on real food.

- Determine your calorie needs.
- Choose the total calories that you are going to eat per day.
- Determine the servings you are allowed from each food group.
- Use your food journal.
- Begin by eating three meals per day.

The three-meals-per-day rhythm works very well for many people, especially those with blood sugar issues. If you need to have a snack between meals in the beginning, that is okay, but cut it out as soon as you can.

Studies show that eating every few hours can help control hunger and equip you to make better food choices throughout the day. However, this is only true if you eat the ideal balance of protein, fat, and carbohydrates. Regularly going below the suggested daily calorie count may actually slow down your progress and increase hunger. If you stick to my plan, you'll avoid this pitfall.

Starting your day off right is important. Most breakfast foods are not balanced—just look at the ingredients. They are probably high in carbohydrates, low in protein, and full of the wrong fats. This combination sets you up for eating way more than you should for the rest of the day.

Month Two: Try an easy FMD.
Restricting food all the time (portion control) affects your weight and hormones differently than restricting food some of the time (intermittent fasting). Let me give you an analogy. If you had a choice, which weather scenario would you prefer:

a) Cloudy and drizzly every day for a week
b) Sunny for five days with two days of heavier rain

Most people would pick option b). Logically, your body has the same preference with calorie restriction. It prefers a few lower calorie days rather than calorie restriction every day.

Here are some results of going on an FMD:

- More weight loss (especially belly fat)
- Greater improvement in insulin sensitivity (a driver of obesity)
- Less muscle loss
- Faster metabolism
- Less chance of weight regain
- Lower levels of ghrelin (the hunger hormone)

FMDs fix weight and hormone problems even faster than calorie restriction. With results like this, you can see why I want you to use this tool. Experiment with it and see what works best for you. Give every plan you try a trial period of several weeks. See Appendix A, Part Six, or 7SystemsPlan.com for more help with FMDs.

The 17-Hour Fast: Simply skip breakfast.
This fast takes little to no effort, but it offers tremendous benefits. Most people aren't hungry in the morning, and it would be very easy for them to skip breakfast. We eat because we have all been taught that breakfast is the most important meal of the day. But if you look at most breakfast studies, they were funded by corporations that make breakfast cereals. That should be a big red flag.

If you do eat breakfast, what often happens? By mid-morning you become hungry, and you eat everything in sight. Has this ever happened to you? We now know that eating "whets the appetite," and the result is that we keep eating. If you don't eat breakfast, you may not experience this mid-morning hunger.

Ghrelin (the hunger hormone) comes in waves throughout the day. It's typically low in the morning and peaks at midday and evening. Unfortunately, you can train your hunger hormone to peak more than it should by eating too frequently and by eating breakfast. There is more and more evidence that skipping breakfast may be the healthier alternative (especially for those who are overweight).

With this method, you consume all your calories in a seven-hour period—ideally between 12 p.m. and 7 p.m. The first week, begin eating at 9 a.m. and keep pushing it back until you get to noon. It is okay to have tea or coffee, but make sure it's black.

It can take up to 60 days for your body to get good at using fat for fuel, so give it time. You can skip your evening meal instead of breakfast, but most people find that more difficult.

The 23-Hour Fast: Skip breakfast and lunch.
With this fast, you follow the 7 Systems Plan one day, then the next day you do not eat until the evening meal. For this meal, eat 500 to 700 calories to make the most progress. I have patients who fast this way three nonconsecutive days a week. Even doing it once a week or a couple of times a month produces visible results.

The 5:2 Fast: Significantly restrict calories two nonconsecutive days per week.
Although I prefer that you continue to restrict calories as suggested on the other five days, this FMD works either way. For two nonconsecutive days, males should limit their calories to 600 per day and females to 500 per day. The principle of this diet is the same as the others: ramp up your body's ability to burn fat for fuel while still supplying adequate nutrition.

Month Three and Beyond: Adjust as you go.
We're all uniquely and wonderfully made. What works great for one person will not work for another. As your awareness increases, make adjustments that fit your body and your goals to find what works best for you.

Quick Recap:

Congratulations on taking a deep dive into your first System— the Structural System. We'll keep exploring the others one at a time. When we're done, each of your seven Systems will be working *with* the others rather than *against* them.

Here's a quick recap of your first System:

- The Structural System has three main parts: bone, muscle, and fat.
- The Structural System has three main functions: to support, move, and store.
- These parts have been compromised by your lifestyle, but they can be fixed.
- You may have bad genes, but they can be silenced.
- Angry fat is a serious problem that you must fix.
- Your body has two fuel sources: calories from your diet and stored fat.
- Your body prefers to run on carbohydrates.
- When you restrict calories or carbohydrates, your body is forced to burn fat.
- You need to optimize your fat-burning ability.
- Healthy calorie restriction and FMDs are powerful tools to speed up your progress toward overall healthiness.

Proven Steps to Fix Your Structural System:

(Check these off as you complete them. Join our free 7 Systems Plan Community for additional support and encouragement: 7SystemsPlan.com.)

☐ Document what you are putting in your body. Start a food journal.

☐ Determine what needs to go; decrease your consumption of ultra-processed food.

☐ Decide to begin the 7 Systems Plan. Stock up on all food groups and start eating more real food.

☐ Change fuel sources by restricting calories.

☐ Discover fasting. Try FMDs and see what works for you.

I suggest you go to the appendix now and read through it for more helpful information. If you have had significant struggles with your weight or health, consider joining my online course (see information at the end of the book) for additional support and help.

Supplements to Support Your Structural System

In the following chapters, I will recommend specific supplements to support each System. If you want to experience results similar to those of my patients, you may want to consider integrating a few products into your diet.

Mary used a functional food to help support her Structural System and lose weight. Functional foods are scientifically formulated products that I have used on countless patients with tremendous results. The 7 Systems Plan works without them, but they will speed up your progress. Dynamic Daily Meal is the best functional food to support your Structural System.

Why do I use functional foods?

- They help Systems return to optimal function more quickly.
- They speed up weight loss.
- They are convenient and easy to use.
- They can be used as a low-cost, low-calorie, tasty meal replacement.
- They help maintain progress.

I provide much more detail at 7SystemsPlan.com and in Appendix A, Part Five.

Structural System Lab Tests

Simple At-Home Test: Waist-to-Hip Ratio

To take these measurements, check the largest measurement at each area, then calculate the ratio by dividing the waist by the hips:

Waist-to-Hip Ratio:		
Male	**Female**	**Health Risk Based Solely on WHR**
0.95 or below	0.80 or below	Low Risk
0.96 to 1.0	0.81 to 0.85	Moderate Risk
1.0+	0.85+	High Risk

Note: If waist and hips are both larger than they should be, this test will not be accurate, but continue to check each month and see the inches melt away.

Bone

DEXA Bone Density
This X-ray technique measures bone density and will give you a rating based on your age, sex, and race. Your results will tell you if you have good bone density, osteopenia, or osteoporosis.

Spinal X-rays
Spinal X-rays are the best way to check for spinal misalignment, disc degeneration, joint degeneration, and many other spinal problems.

Fat and Muscle

Best Test: Bioimpedance Analysis (BIA)
This simple, inexpensive test can be performed by a functional medicine doctor. Over 100 independent studies conducted over the past 20 years have demonstrated that BIA can provide an accurate and clinically useful assessment of body composition.

BIA is performed with the help of a sophisticated computerized analysis. First, measurements are taken with the bioimpedance device. The BIA calculates your body compartments using a gentle electrical current passed through your hands and feet. Optimal body fat ranges from 15% to 25% for women and 10% to 20% for men. Optimal ranges for muscle, fat, and additional information will be given on the test report. See 7SystemsPlan.com for more information.

2

The Digestive System Gut and Brain

Put your second brain to work—the right way.

Startling Facts

- An estimated 60 million Americans have a digestive disease.[1]
- Americans spend $2 billion a year on over-the-counter heartburn medications alone.[2]
- Digestive problems are some of the top issues that send people to their doctors.[3]
- The Digestive System and brain have a unique relationship and constantly communicate. The health of one has a tremendous effect on the other.[4,5]

> "Ever 'gone with your gut' to make a decision or felt 'butterflies in your stomach' when nervous? You're likely getting signals from an unexpected source:
> *your second* brain."
> —Johns Hopkins Medicine

Let's imagine that your Structural System is now supported with real food. Now the Digestive System's job is to break the food down into smaller materials that can enter the bloodstream.

A Brief Introduction to The Digestive System

The Digestive System is also referred to as the gut, gastrointestinal tract, or GI tract, but don't get lost in semantics. Most people know the basic digestive process.

First, you chew food. Next, it goes into the stomach where acids and enzymes are dumped in. Then, the food passes through the small intestine where nutrients are extracted. And finally, the waste goes to the colon and out of the body.

This is what we have been taught.

But this summary leaves out a vital player—the brain. Once we understand the relationship between the Digestive System and the brain, a brand new world opens up, and we are closer to solving weight loss problems and health issues.

The brain is considered part of the Digestive System because it impacts why we eat, when we eat, and how we eat. Digestion, cravings, and addictions originate in both the brain and gut. If you ignore either, you'll struggle with losing weight and getting healthy. But the opposite is true too—if you get them working together properly, then achieving your health goals will be much easier.

Ready to take a deeper dive into the Digestive System?

7 Signs That Your Digestive System Is Working Against You:

1. Difficulty keeping your weight under control, even though you watch your diet
2. Alternating between constipation and urgency
3. Indigestion, intestinal gas, bloating, gastric reflux, or bad breath
4. Stomach or intestinal pain

5. Headaches
6. Food allergies or sensitivities
7. Depression or mood swings

Meet Jennifer

Jennifer appeared a little uncomfortable as she sat down in my office and began to share her story. "I have been diagnosed with irritable bowel syndrome (IBS). I have acid reflux, frequent gas, bloating, and pain in my abdomen. This has been going on for over 10 years and seems to be getting worse." She had been taking prescriptions for acid reflux and pain medication, but with little benefit.

She was overweight, moody, irritable, and at times, even depressed. She had also been diagnosed with psoriasis—an autoimmune condition that caused plaque to form on her skin. Her lab tests showed mild obesity, elevated inflammatory markers, and a vitamin D deficiency (often linked to an autoimmune disease).

Her health history revealed a poor diet lacking vegetables and full of junk food, two diet soft drinks per day, and use of antibiotics the prior year for bronchitis.

We needed to face the facts and address her Digestive System. We began by giving her a high dose of vitamin D3, probiotics, a functional food, and the 7 Systems Plan.

After three months, she achieved her ideal weight. She no longer suffered from acid reflux and was off her prescriptions. All her GI distress had disappeared. A second round of tests revealed normal levels of Vitamin D, and her inflammatory markers were normal. Even her psoriasis was on the fast track to being fully resolved. She had moved from feeling depressed and miserable to enjoying life again and was all smiles at her last visit to my office.

Why Your Digestive System Is Working Against You

If you are going to lose more weight, start feeling better, and slow down the aging process, you need to understand two things: how your Digestive System works and how to get it functioning properly.

The Digestive System has a lot more going on than we once thought. Out of it flows a wide array of physiological processes including your immune function, detoxification, inflammation, neurotransmitter and vitamin production, nutrient absorption, hunger and fullness signals, and the digestion of carbohydrates, protein, and fat. When these processes break down, it results in chronic problems with allergies, asthma, ADHD, cancer, diabetes, dementia, and a myriad of other health issues.

Hardly a week passes without a new study confirming the importance of your microbiome (gut bacteria). We now know that it affects your weight, mood, libido, metabolism, immunity, and even your perception of the world and clarity of your thoughts. It plays a role in whether you are overweight or thin, energetic or tired. It is a key part of the Digestive System, which influences so many other Systems and determines how you feel emotionally and physically. Unfortunately, the modern lifestyle has destroyed our healthy gut microbiome, leaving us vulnerable.

The good news is that most problems with this System are reversible. If you know your gut's vital role within your body and how it functions, you can make a few adjustments and eliminate weight gain, fix Defense System malfunctions, eradicate sickness, improve mental health issues, and reverse aging.

Because your "head brain" and "gut brain" work together, we'll begin by addressing your head brain. We'll figure out the obstacles that stand in your way (including habits and addictions) that keep you from having the health you want. Also, you'll discover how to trick your body out of hunger, cravings, and social pressures.

The Brain

The digestive process begins before you even put food into your mouth. Can you relate to this scenario? You sit down and look at a good meal. Suddenly, your mouth begins to water.

Why?

Your brain starts the digestive process by sending signals to your Digestive System. When you eat mindlessly or while distracted, your brain is less involved in the process, impairing the System's proper function.

Food manufacturers know that you tend to shop and eat mindlessly. As a result, they produce food that is engineered to addict you. Obviously, they want you to buy their product again and again.

The more you eat this unhealthy food, the less your taste buds enjoy the taste of real food. This creates a harmful cycle, driving you to eat more and more bad food. In a way, we're all being brainwashed, or—better said—"tastewashed."

Some foods even have the ability to stimulate the "feel good" sensors in your brain. Think about it. Have you ever seen someone's eyes roll back in delight when consuming junk food? Addictions develop because it will take more and more of this food to give you that initial buzz (just like illegal drugs).

Thankfully, this toxic cycle can be broken.

Do this:

- *Decrease junk food.* Good food will taste better, and the sooner you replace junk food with healthy food, the sooner your brain can reset itself. Your taste buds and brain are reprogrammable.
- *Eat mindfully.* By becoming aware of what you're eating, you'll be mentally prepared for better digestion. You want your meals to register with your brain. People who eat while distracted (watching TV, at a sports game, etc.) can eat up to 50% more![6]
- *Pause before eating.* Wait for one to two minutes before you begin. Look at the food. Smell the food. Think about what you are about to eat.

The Mouth

Up to one-third of digestion takes place in your mouth. If food is not adequately chewed, it's much more difficult for the rest of the Digestive System to do its job. Many people (particularly those who are overweight) do not chew food adequately.

Real food contains many natural enzymes. If you have ever bruised a piece of fruit, you have seen the enzymes begin to digest it as it turns brown. These same enzymes aid your digestion. Eating real food and chewing properly can result in up to 70% of digestion being done before the stomach even gets involved.

Do this:

- *Slow down and enjoy the food you eat.* Put your fork down between bites. Pace yourself with the slowest eater at the table. Chew each bite at least 20 times.
- *Eat real food.*

The Esophagus

When you stop and think about it, your body is an amazing creation. Look no further than the esophagus, and you'll see what I mean.

The esophagus is an eight-inch tube that moves food and liquid in waves into the stomach. Since acid in the stomach can damage the esophagus, there is a valve, or sphincter, to hold the acid in the stomach and keep it from coming back up. The valve is designed to contract when your brain knows you're eating. If this valve doesn't close, acid from the stomach can get up the esophagus into the trachea, possibly affecting the lungs.

If you suffer from heartburn (acid in the esophagus), you may be using antacids or proton pump inhibitors (PPIs) to neutralize or stop the production of acid. Although this relieves the symptoms, it brings on a host of other health problems, including weight gain. You cannot digest food without stomach acid. In a recent study, PPIs were linked to 7.7 pounds of weight gain in 2.2 years. PPIs also destroy good gut bacteria, creating additional intestinal issues. In addition, a study in *The Journal of the American Medical Association* (*JAMA*) also reported a strong statistical link between regular use of these medications and Alzheimer's.[7]

Do this:

- *Determine the cause of your reflux.* Some of the most common catalysts are eating too large of a meal, fatty foods, acidic juices, fruit, alcohol, and caffeine. You can also experience symptoms from eating while distracted, lying down after eating, not having enough stomach acid, taking antacids or PPIs, or carrying too much belly fat. See 7SystemsPlan.com to download a proven plan I use to help many of my patients get off PPIs.

The Stomach

The stomach is like a complex washing machine—combining acids, enzymes (pepsinogen and lipase), and fluids with the food you eat and then mixing it around and around. Ideally, your stomach should produce two quarts of this liquid per day to break down your food. Your body needs these acids and enzymes to absorb certain micronutrients like calcium, folate, B12, and iron. Stomach acid also kills bad bacteria that cause illness. These bacteria should not get into your small intestine.

Stomach acid is essential. Hypochlorhydria (lack of stomach acid) becomes a common problem as people age. Warning signs include bloating, belching, and flatulence immediately after meals. Other signs include heartburn (often incorrectly thought to be a result of too much stomach acid), indigestion, and undigested food in stools, to name a few. Undigested food is a serious issue because it can damage the intestinal tract.

A strong protective layer called mucin prevents the acid from harming your stomach and GI tract. Good bacteria in your GI tract keep the mucin in working condition. If this mucin layer is damaged, the lining becomes vulnerable to erosion. This layer can be weakened by the frequent use of over-the-counter pain medicine (NSAIDs). Up to 50% of all people taking NSAIDs injure their Digestive System.[8]

Stretch receptors in your stomach communicate with your brain. Your stomach measures the volume, pH, and consistency of your food and then signals the brain and other organs, telling them what to do next. When your stomach is full, it tells your brain that you have eaten enough. This triggers a decrease in appetite and, naturally, most people stop eating.

It is important to know that these receptors measure *volume*, not *calories*. Until you meet your stomach's volume need, the appetite sensor will stay on, no matter how many calories you've eaten!

Think about this: You can feel full just by drinking a large glass of water. Although there are no calories, the volume "fills" you up. Unfortunately, today there are many calorie-dense, low-volume foods available. Although they don't take up much space, they pack a powerful punch of calories. These foods don't trip your volume sensor to make you feel full; they lead to faster weight gain because it's hard to stop eating them. Thankfully, the 7 Systems Plan solves this problem.

The average stomach holds about one liter of fluid, no matter your weight. You do, however, have the ability to enlarge your stomach, increasing the amount of food you can eat at one time. In the 2015 Nathan's Hot Dog Eating Contest, the winner ate 70 hot dogs with buns in 10 minutes. This type of unhealthy feat can only be done by severely enlarging your stomach.

Do this:

- *Treat your hypochlorhydria.* If you have bloating, belching, and flatulence immediately after meals, take a couple of betaine hydrochloride pills with your meal and see if it resolves the symptoms.
- *Use as few NSAIDs as possible.* All prescriptions and over-the-counter medications have side effects.
- *Trip your stomach volume sensor.* Stop eating calorie-dense, low-volume foods and follow the 7 Systems Plan.

- *Shrink your stomach.* Studies have shown that by eating smaller meals for four weeks, you can reduce your stomach capacity. After one month, you will feel full with less food.

The Small Intestine

When food in the stomach is ready, it is released to move into the small intestinal tract. As complex and important as your stomach is, the small intestine is even more intricate and has more work to do.

This 20-foot-long tube is responsible for continuing the breakdown of food into small molecules, getting nutrients into the bloodstream and keeping harmful material out. In the intestine, there is only a one-cell-thick layer separating material in the gut from the bloodstream. Therefore, the health and function of these intestinal cells and the mucin layer protecting them is critical.

The liver assists the small intestine in this process by producing bile that breaks down fats. It does this via the gallbladder. The pancreas then adds a fluid full of enzymes (including proteases, lipase, and amylase), eight cups per day, to break down protein, fats, and carbohydrates.

Although the other organs get most of the attention, the true MVP of this game is the villi. You need more than the 20 feet of small intestine to absorb nutrients, so lining the intestinal tract are millions of small, thumb-like structures called villi. With this new player, the surface area increases to the size of a football field.

Cells on the tips of the villi secrete enzymes that help break down milk, sugar, and other nutrients. If you eat fruits and vegetables, they contain natural enzymes that aid villi in the digestive process. Most people don't know that the tips of these villi can be shaved off or damaged by lack of stomach acid (use of PPIs), undigested food, diarrhea, food allergies, and disease. This will severely hinder the digestion and absorption of nutrients. Having the wrong bacteria in your gut can also damage the protective mucin layer over the villi, causing further problems.

Failure to digest and absorb nutrients is a common break-down within the Digestive System. But with a few tweaks—like restoring good bacteria through probiotics and adding enzymes contained in real foods—these nutrients have a much better chance of being digested and absorbed.

Interesting Fact

You have a nutrient sensor in your gut that signals the brain when enough nutrients have been consumed. Protein and healthy fats trigger the release of hormones that turn off hunger. If you don't consume these nutrients, your gut can tell the brain to send out hunger signals in hopes that you will eat the nutrients that are needed.

The SAD (standard American diet) is missing many essential nutrients, so our brains keep asking for food via hunger pangs and cravings. By eating the high-nutrient diet found within *7 Systems Plan*, you can silence these hunger signals.

In the crevices between these thumb-like projections resides 70% of your Defense System—Peyer's patches. Your body must be able to defend against hostile elements wanting to get in. If you have a healthy gut with tight junctions between the intestinal cells, it makes the Defense System's job a lot easier. If not, undigested food, harmful material, and bad bacteria can enter your bloodstream and cause an immune response. When this happens, it can trigger a chronic inflammatory process that affects your entire body. Many chronic and autoimmune diseases originate here. We'll unpack more of this in Chapter Six.

Good bacteria in the gut thrive on fiber and provide protection. They preserve and protect the mucin layer, producing vitamins, extracting energy from food, and protecting cells from carcinogenic changes. Lack of fiber, excess sugar, and bad fats increase bad bacteria. Every day, your food choices determine which bacteria will thrive and which will die.

Remember, your gut has a considerable influence on what, why, and when you eat, so it is important that it functions correctly.

Digestion, mood, appetite, cravings, and addictions all have their origin here. As a result, you cannot neglect your gut if you want to lose weight and be healthy. When it comes to losing weight, your "gut-set" may be more important than your mindset.

Do this:

- *Take care of your mucin layer.* Repair the protective mucin layer by eating real food full of natural enzymes and taking probiotics.
- *Eat fiber-rich foods.* The prebiotics in these foods will feed the good bacteria in your Digestive System.

The Large Intestine

The large intestine, also known as the colon, plays a critical role in the Digestive System. It's responsible for absorbing water to keep the body fluid balance correct and moving material to the rectum to be stored and excreted.

It should take 12–30 hours for food to make its journey from the mouth to the toilet. If it takes any longer than that, toxins will be absorbed by the colon.

Do this:

- *Stay regular by having daily bowel movements.* We will talk more about this in Chapter Seven: The Detox System.

The Gut-Brain Connection

As you now know, the Digestive System and the brain are intricately connected. Although this is interesting information, you'll never experience transformation unless you know how to optimize this knowledge.

Both the gut and the brain were created from identical tissue during your development. The brain doesn't have this unique connection with any other System, and the gut is the only System that has its own brain.

We often think of the brain as the control center of the body, but your gut sends far more information to your brain than your brain sends to your gut. Communication takes place through electrical impulses through billions of neurons and a highway of chemicals and hormones.

For years we've known that the brain sends signals to the gut. Terms like "butterflies in your stomach" or "instant diarrhea" reflect this understanding. However, in recent years, we've observed how the gut constantly communicates with the brain by the vagus nerve. It is the longest nerve from the brain and has the widest distribution of any nerve in the body, branching out to the entire Digestive System. This is one way the brain and Digestive System communicate, and it is important to know that 90% of all the signals passing along this nerve are traveling from the gut to the brain, not vice versa.

It may surprise you to know that your gut bacteria are the largest source of these signals. Good bacteria produce vitamins, aid in digestion, rebuild the protective mucin layer, turn off the hunger hormone, decrease inflammation, and signal the brain to make good food choices. Your brain depends upon this information to keep your body healthy. These bacteria tell your brain what food you should eat and when you should eat it. The bacteria in your gut can literally control your brain.

The idea that gut bacteria have a tremendous influence on your health is not a new concept. In 1907, Élie Metchnikoff wrote in *The Prolongation of Life* that disease and aging come from the bacteria in your gut.[9] In the last 10 years, the research supporting this has exploded, and now it is a proven fact.

Your gut bacteria have been compared to a rainforest—an entire ecosystem of living organisms dwelling in a delicate balance. If a rainforest is healthy and strong, life thrives. The same is true for the human body.

Unfortunately, many things in our world today upset this balance. Taking one course of antibiotics can wipe out your entire "ecosystem" for two years. Imagine a fire destroying an entire rainforest—it takes a long time for it to recover.

When good bacteria have been eliminated, bad bacteria, yeast, fungus, and molds take over. Remember, microbes tell the brain what food to consume. Here's a little secret: Bad bacteria send signals through the bloodstream and the vagus nerve to your brain to eat more junk food, saturated fat, and sugar. They influence your food choices and weight in a negative way. You can have trillions of these bad bacteria signaling your brain to eat the type of food that feeds them.

As they multiply, the bad bacteria begin spilling out of your gut and affecting other Systems. The result is inflammation, infections, skin problems, gas, bloating, indigestion, and (most significantly) weight gain.

Unfortunately, antibiotics aren't the only problem. Chlorinated drinking water, processed meat containing antibiotics, statin drugs, antidepressants, pain pills, acid reflux medication, artificial sweeteners, lack of fiber, too much sugar, and bad fat can also devastate your internal rainforest.

A study at Duke University in 2008 showed that the use of artificial sweeteners kills off beneficial microbes in your gut. Artificial sweeteners used in diet soft drinks are most likely the reason that diet soft drinks cause weight gain.[10]

How to Get Your Digestive System Working for You

Just as with the Structure System, the Digestive System is either working for you or against you. If you can get this System on your side, then losing weight, feeling better, and looking younger will become much easier.

Let's get your gut and brain working for you again.

Step 1: Fix your rainforest.

First, you must stop killing off your good bacteria. Avoid the things that damage them.

Second, it is extremely helpful to continually put good bacteria (probiotics) back into your gut. Probiotic supplements and fermented foods can help with this. But just putting the bacteria back into the gut is like planting a tree and never watering or fertilizing it. These bacteria can only live about two weeks without the right food.

The third part of the process is to feed the beneficial bacteria with prebiotics. Good bacteria thrive on fiber. This is one of the many reasons the 7 Systems Plan recommends eating more fruits and vegetables—they help sustain your microbiome.

If you have significant problems with this System, you may need to do a gut restart with a couple of products found at 7SystemsPlan.com. While no one can really start over with all-new bacteria, nutritional science is making it easier than ever to come close to it.

Probiotics and Weight Management
Much evidence supports the use of probiotics for the management of body weight. Here is what we know at this time:

- Lean people have different bacteria and a greater variety of bacteria in their gut than obese people.
- The greater the diversity of good bacteria, the thinner and healthier you will be.
- Putting good bacteria into obese people leads to weight loss and other health benefits.

Remain vigilant. According to the World Health Organization (WHO), not all probiotics are the same. The health benefits of probiotics are genus, species, and strain specific, and probiotics should be chosen based on the desired health benefits.[11]

Clinical evidence now supports the use of B420 (*Bifidobacterium animalis ssp. Lactis*) for body weight and body fat mass regulation as well as GI health and cardiometabolic health.[12]

The B420 in one of my recommended products, UltraBiotic Integrity, has been shown to make you

- Less hungry (by increasing short-chain fatty acids)
- Eat less (by reducing your caloric intake by 300 calories)
- Have lower blood sugar (by improving glucose metabolism)
- Thinner (by reducing your waist circumference)
- Gain less weight (by reducing fat mass)
- Healthier (by reducing intestinal permeability—leaky gut)
- Decrease inflammation (by reducing levels of hs-CRP)[13]

Prebiotics and Weight Management
Following the 7 Systems Plan will supply the fiber necessary to feed good bacteria and help them multiply. At the end of this chapter, I will discuss a medical product that is great for weight loss, GI healing, and feeding beneficial bacteria.

Do this:

- *Make healthy food choices.* Change your eating habits and focus on how you feel so much better *today*—you will.
- *Change your gut and your mind.* Your appetite and the amount of food you need is largely controlled by your gut and your brain. Therefore, losing weight is mainly a gut and mind game. If you can change your gut and your mind, then you can change your body.

Step 2: Know why you are hungry.

Many patients struggle on the path toward healthiness because they feel hungry all the time. They know they want to change, but relying on willpower alone is not a plan. They need a stronger strategy.

You have been programmed by culture and tradition to assign meaning to food and occasions surrounding food. No wonder most of us lose sight of the very reason we eat: to get essential fuel and nutrients needed to function and rebuild our bodies. Many people think that food is all about taste—that we should only eat things that taste great. This is dangerous because you can warp your taste buds so that your body wants more of the wrong food.

If you saw *Super Size Me*, you witnessed someone who was initially repulsed by junk food become addicted and crave more in just 30 days. Eating these foods elevates the neurotransmitter dopamine, which then binds to its receptor site in the brain, making you feel good and want more. The reward and pleasure pathways in the brain can be hijacked by these foods, causing addictions identical to those of an alcoholic or drug abuser.

Have you ever walked by a box of donuts at work and felt your mouth begin to water? Hunger can be a learned behavior, triggered by physiological stimuli and psychological stimuli (Pavlov's dog). The good news is that we can change both of these, and I will give you lots of tools to do this.

Physiological Hunger Sources
1. Hormonal Hunger (Ghrelin)
You might remember this from Chapter One, but here is a bit more information. Ghrelin is produced in waves throughout the day, and it subsides after the initial wave, whether you eat or not. If you ignore it or simply have a warm drink, it will go away. Women tend to have larger waves than men, and since larger waves mean more hunger, this may explain why women have more food addiction problems. Following the 7 Systems Plan will help you train your hunger hormone and make it much weaker.

2. Fat Cell Hunger
Your fat cells can make you hungry in several ways. Remember, fat cells are like selfish children stealing your calories. They also send out bad messenger molecules telling your body to eat and store more fat. The more fat you have, the more of a problem this becomes. Chances are you have some working against you right now. In time, you'll weaken their power and then eliminate it. See "How to Get Leptin Working for You" in Chapter Five.

3. Bad Bacteria Hunger

Bad bacteria signal the brain to eat more junk food. Changing your microbes and following the 7 Systems Plan will fix this problem.

In one study, the gut bacteria from an obese person was put into a mouse. The gut bacteria from a person of normal weight was put into a different mouse. The obese person's bacteria caused a normal mouse to become obese while the other did not. Overweight people have the wrong bacteria in their Digestive System working against them.[14]

4. Volume and Nutrient Deficiency Hunger

The high-calorie, low-volume food you eat may not be tripping the stretch receptors in your stomach. Your diet may also be low in micronutrients, protein, and heathy fats. Your body has powerful hormones that turn off hunger, but they need these nutrients in order to work.

5. Low Blood Sugar Hunger

If you make poor food choices (eat bad carbohydrates), your blood sugar can swing from high to low, triggering hunger and cravings. Many of my patients who begin the 7 Systems Plan are carbohydrate addicts. You'll achieve more of your goals by avoiding bad carbohydrates.

6. Dehydration Hunger

Has this ever happened to you? You eat a nice meal, and 30 minutes later, you're hungry. Biologically speaking, this is impossible. You're probably getting a thirst signal—not a hunger one. They can feel the same. Hunger is often the first sensation people get when their body is low on water. As people age, their thirst signal gets weaker and is often confused with their hunger signal. To solve this problem, try drinking a big glass of water and wait 20 minutes. If you're no longer hungry, you've identified and eliminated the false signal.

7. Food Addiction Hunger
This is no longer a theory. Refined and processed foods known as hyper-palatables are combinations of sugary, fatty, and salty foods. They can cause addictions by giving you a buzz (good feeling). Make no mistake—this is a powerful feeling. We will cover breaking this addiction in detail in Chapter Five—the Communication System.

8. Stress Hunger
Do you eat when you're stressed? Elevated hormones (cortisol) can cause you to crave foods high in sugar and fat (most common in females). These bad foods give you a short burst of comfort but add to your problems.

Psychological Hunger Sources
To help with psychological hunger, do not eat

- *For comfort*—Many people were raised on so-called comfort foods.
- *Family style*—Setting the food on the table will cause you to eat 20-30% more. Leave the food on the counter.
- *Off large plates*—This gives your brain the perception that you are being deprived because the plate is not full. Using smaller plates will help you consume 22% less.
- *Out with others too much*—When you eat out with others, you tend to eat more. When you eat with one friend, you consume 35% more calories. If there are four of you eating, you may consume 75% more calories. At a big event, with seven or more people, you may consume 95% more calories!
- *From a bag or box*—This is never a good idea because you will eat much more than you would otherwise.
- *While distracted*—You will eat 10% more. To make matters worse, you will eat 25% more at your next meal. Taken together, mindless eating can boost what you eat by up to 50%! If you remove the distractions, look at your food, and smell your food, you will eat 10% less at your next meal.

Do this:

- *Think of real food as an antidepressant, because it is.* The psychology behind food addictions and cravings is a big deal. We'll unpack this later on in Chapter Five, but for now, spend a moment focusing on why you have been eating the wrong food.
- *Think of eating to live, not living to eat.* Think of real food as medicine, not comfort. This will give you much more energy. If you're a food addict or carbohydrate addict, be prepared—you may have some withdrawal symptoms for the first one or two weeks. But after a short amount of time, you will feel much better. Check out The 7 Systems Online Course for more information and help with food addictions.

Step 3: Realize that, without help, your willpower will fail you.

Remember Jennifer? Over a three-month period, she lost weight, regained her health, got a younger body, and felt great.

At the same time, a middle-aged woman named Debbie contacted me about her weight problems and type 2 diabetes. Both of these problems were progressively getting worse. She knew that taking more and more drugs was not the answer, but that was what she had been doing. She wanted to change her unhealthy lifestyle but just didn't have enough willpower.

In the end, one of these women was successful, and one was not. The difference? One woman understood how to add helpers to her willpower, and the other didn't.

Meet Mr. Will Power.

Imagine a "tug of war" in which you're trying to win out over poor health and weight gain. Since you're struggling, you recruit Mr. Will Power. Although he looks impressive, he's quite weak and vastly outnumbered by the opposing side.

Having worked with thousands of people over the years, I often meet patients who initially think they just need more willpower in order to lose weight and regain health. This is a recipe for failure.

One of the problems is that, up until now, you've been blind-folded and ignorant of what is pulling against you and your willpower. These opponents are strong and numerous.

Now imagine that same tug of war, but this time you can identify and eliminate the things pulling against you and even get them pulling for you. Obviously, this makes it much easier to win. Now you have a team to defeat your weight and health problems.

I'm going to help you win the battle for good.

Do this:

- *Take the blindfold off.*
- *Identify the opponents that are pulling against you.*
- *Convert them into helpers to pull with you.*

Step 4: Stack your side for success.

No one has enough willpower to make the right decisions all the time. The good news is, you can "stack your side" by giving Mr. Will Power some helpers. The more you can add, the greater success you will have.

Helper #1: Desire

I ask everyone I work with one key question: "Do you want to change your health?" This sounds pretty straightforward, but psychologists agree that the desire to change is essential before any change is possible. The good news is the fact that you're reading this book tells me you have a desire to change. But you need to pinpoint the "why" behind your desire.

Knowing your why will help you stay motivated and keep you on track in difficult times.

Do this:
On a 3x5 card, list out what you want to do and why you want to do it. Here are some examples:

- "I want to lose weight so that I have more energy to do my job."
- "I want to get healthy so that I can get off my prescription medication."
- "I want to be thin so that I will feel better about how I look."

Make your list and look at it each time you struggle.

Helper #2: Skills

To make weight loss easier, you need to acquire new skills and abilities. Reading this book is a great start. Studies show that the more educated a person is, the better health choices they make. Invest time in becoming a health and weight expert.

In my clinic, I teach weekly classes, which are also available in an online course. The patients who lose weight and fix their Systems the fastest are those who attend the classes, take notes, and apply what they have learned to their own lives.

Do this:

- Finish reading this book.
- Visit 7SystemsPlan.com and check out my online course and additional resources that will help you on your journey toward health.

Helper #3: Cheering Section

In my clinic, every time a patient loses another 10 pounds, we have them come up to the front of the class and take a picture. We cheer and clap to encourage them. My patients have friends supporting them. Success rates are even higher when my patients have their friends or spouse working together with them on their health goals. Make sure you surround yourself with others who will encourage you.

Be aware. You may need to distance yourself from people who try to sabotage you. You may need to stop eating out with them. Refrain from putting yourself in a situation where you're tempted by behavior that doesn't match your goals.

Do this:

- Identify the people hindering your progress and distance yourself if necessary.
- Stack your side by finding friends who will support and cheer you on.
- Ask friends for a verbal commitment to support you.

Helper #4: Coach

Coaches help us excel at many different things. You might have a pastor who serves as a spiritual coach or a financial advisor who serves as your financial coach.

One of the most important coaches you can have is a health coach. This person will help you develop a plan to achieve health goals. This coach will help you monitor progress and encourage you to keep going. With your permission, I would be honored to serve as your health coach. With this book, I will help you develop a program that works for you.

Do this:

- Continue to read this book and develop your plan
- For more information and additional support, visit 7SystemsPlan.com.
- Find someone who will hold you accountable weekly.

Helper #5: Rewards and Incentives

Ask any child or adult—rewards and incentives are powerful motivators. Surprisingly, they do not have to be extravagant. It's essential that you reward yourself for milestones, big or small. Every little success, when multiplied, adds up to bigger successes. Here are some milestone examples:

- When you exercise 20 minutes longer than you used to be able to

- When you're 10 pounds lighter
- When that smaller size fits you
- When you realize that you have gone a month without that particular tempting treat and you do not feel like you need it anymore

These are all successes worth celebrating.

These rewards must be something other than food. You need to learn how reward yourself with things other than food or treats.

Incentives shape behavior. Patients who have an event coming up in a few months, like a son or daughter's wedding, have greater success achieving their weight-loss goals. This is an example of what I call the Event Incentive.

Event + Goal = Incentive

Do this:

- Try to link your health goals with an important event (a wedding, high school reunion, trip, or even your birthday).
- Once you hit a small goal, reward yourself. Put a card on the refrigerator with your goal and add a star each time you hit 10 more pounds off. When you hit a big goal (lost 30 pounds), buy some new clothes, go on a trip, buy a treadmill, get your hair colored, or do something to make yourself look even younger.

Helper #6: Health-Friendly Environment

I have a confession. I can have ice cream in the freezer for months and never touch it. But if there are peanut M&M's in the cupboard, they will not last long.

What fits in that category for you? What do you need to remove from your house? If you're trying to lose weight and your house is filled with junk food, chances are you will fail.

Do this:

- Purge your house. Throw out everything that sabotages your success. Toss it out. Don't eat it up.
- The house may not be the only place you need to purge. Some people have junk food at their workstations or in their car or purse. Remove everything that makes it more difficult for you to succeed.
- As you remove bad food and bad habits, replace them with good ones to increase your success significantly.

I provide a worksheet for you in Appendix A, Part Four, to help you develop your success team.

Let's revisit Jennifer and Debbie.

Jennifer wanted to get her health back. As a result, she identified the things pulling against her and eliminated many of them. Next, she stacked her side. On 3x5 cards, she listed the reasons she wanted to get healthy. She started attending my class each week with her husband, desiring to learn something new.

She also let her friends know what she was doing and asked them to encourage her. She was accountable to me as her coach, and I cheered her on when she made progress. She got all the junk food out of her house and planned to buy some new clothes when she achieved her health goals. By eliminating the things pulling against her and stacking her side, she ultimately won the fight.

Debbie also wanted to lose weight and get healthy. She came in for testing and recommendations. However, she neither identified the opponents nor acquired new skills and abilities. Her husband was supportive, but he did not change his diet. As a result, she had no accountability or rewards in place. At work, junk food was readily available.

To no one's surprise, she abandoned the program. Unfortunately, her diabetes got worse, resulting in weeks in the hospital. Keep reading, though—even this story has a happy ending.

Quick Recap:

- Your gut and brain have a unique relationship and communicate constantly.
- Your Digestive System is the root of most disease.
- You must use your mind when you eat.
- Adequately chewing your food aids in digestion.
- There are healthy things you can do to eliminate acid reflux.
- Long-term use of antacids and PPIs can have serious health consequences.
- Your stomach has a volume sensor, not a calorie sensor.
- Your gut's health is of paramount importance to all your Systems.
- You should experience bowel movements on a daily basis.
- There are many causes of hunger. Identify yours.
- Depending on willpower alone will lead to failure.

Proven Steps to Fix Your Digestive System:

(Check these off as you complete them. Join our free 7 Systems Plan Community for additional support and encouragement: 7SystemsPlan.com.)

- ☐ Fix your gut and keep the gut–brain connection healthy. Follow the 7 Systems Plan.

- ☐ Know why you are hungry. Identify the hunger sources that plague you.

- ☐ Support your gut microbiome. Stop killing the good bacteria; add probiotics and feed them.

- ☐ Recruit the six willpower helpers. Eliminate the things pulling against you, and start stacking your side for success.

Supplements to Support Your Digestive System

A healthy Digestive System requires that you have good bacteria and that you feed them. This can be achieved by following the 7 Systems Plan. For additional support, use UltraBiotic Integrity and a prebiotic functional food (Dynamic GI Restore) as Jennifer did. See Appendix A, Part Five, for more information.

Digestive System Lab Tests

Simple At-Home Test: Evaluate Your Stool

- Do you have daily, well-formed bowel movements? They should be tan in color, not too hard and not too liquid.
- You should not have gut pain or discomfort and not need antacids, anti-inflammatories, or laxative medications.

Stomach Acid Production

Mix 1/4 teaspoon of baking soda with five ounces of cold water and drink it first thing in the morning, before eating or drinking anything else. The combination of baking soda and hydrochloric acid in your stomach creates carbon dioxide gas, causing you to belch.

Time yourself for five minutes to see how long it takes to form enough gas in your stomach to belch. Belching in two to three minutes is normal. Earlier and repeated belching indicates an excess of acid. If you do not belch after five minutes, most likely you do not produce enough acid.

Bowel Transit Time

Get some charcoal tablets from the health food store. Take some in the morning, and see how many hours it takes to show up dark in your stool. The next day, take some at noon, and the next day at dinner.

This test enables you to see how long it takes for food to pass through your Digestive System. The hours it takes will be your bowel transit time. The ideal time is 12–24 hours. A shorter time may indicate malabsorption problems, and a longer time suggests a sluggish colon.

Additional Tests

Visit 7SystemsPlan.com for information on more tests to evaluate your Digestive System. These tests can reveal parasites, bad bacteria, leaky gut, and the balance of beneficial bacteria.

3

The Delivery System Nutrients and How They Are Delivered

Make sure the goods arrive safely and on time.

Startling Facts

- Every 42 seconds, someone in America has a heart attack.[1]
- Every 60 seconds, someone dies from a heart-related disease.[2]
- If you are over 40 years of age, the chance of you having an arterial disease is 95%.
- As of 2015, 50% of all Americans have diabetes or prediabetes.[3]
- At the current rate, 1 in 3 children will have diabetes, and almost 100% will have fatty streaks in their arteries by age 10.[4,5]

"The food you eat can be either the safest and most powerful
form of medicine or the slowest form of poison."
—Ann Wigmore

Let's imagine that your other two Systems have been working correctly up to this point:

- Your Structural System is supported with real food.
- Your Digestive System broke the food down into small nutrients.

And now, the nutrients have to be delivered to the cells for their use. This is where your Delivery System takes over.

A Brief Introduction to The Delivery System

No matter how nutritious your food is, you won't get any benefit if the nutrients never get where they need to go. After food is consumed, it moves through your Digestive System and the nutrients are extracted. They wait here to "catch a ride" to your muscles, organs, and tissues. This is where the Delivery System comes in.

Nutrients fall into two groups: macronutrients and micronutrients. The macronutrients are larger molecules measured in grams. They are sorted even further into three groups: fat, protein, and carbohydrates. The micronutrients are smaller molecules measured in milligrams. They fall into two basic groups: vitamins and minerals. Vitamins are further sorted into two groups: fat-soluble and water-soluble.

Each group of nutrients is transported differently. Most macronutrients and micronutrients have a carrier that picks them up and delivers them where they're needed. These carriers must work right for this System to function correctly.

Macronutrients:	Micronutrients:
Larger, Measured in Grams	Smaller, Measured in Milligrams
Fats, Proteins, Carbohydrates	Vitamins (Fat/Water-Soluble), Minerals

Knowing how your Delivery System works, what is not working, and then making changes to get it functioning properly will help you fix this System, lose weight, heal and prevent diseases, and reverse aging for good.

It all starts with changing the nutrients that you deliver to your cells. When you do this, your body starts working for you, not against you. Problems in the Delivery System (resulting in type 2 diabetes and heart disease) often decrease or go away completely.

Since what you eat determines how well the Delivery System works, you will never fix this System unless you start consuming the right macronutrients and micronutrients. No prescription drug, pill, or vitamin alone will fix this System. The fix can be easy and fast (you may see results within a few weeks) if you understand and start practicing the 7 Systems Plan.

7 Signs That Your Delivery System Is Working Against You:

1. Weight gain
2. Brain fog or feeling sleepy after meals
3. High blood pressure, LDL cholesterol, or triglycerides
4. Loss of muscle
5. High blood sugar
6. Decreased kidney function
7. Heart or blood vessel problems or use of statin drugs

Meet Ray

When Ray first came to me, I immediately noticed the anxiety written all over his face. I saw the typical signs of fear: slumped shoulders, downcast eyes, and fidgeting hands.

He confided that he'd had heart bypass surgery several years ago, and now an angiogram confirmed that the artery was plugged again. Clearly, he did not want to go through surgery again, but his condition was severe. His heart problem was the result of a poor diet and a malfunctioning Delivery System.

He had high blood pressure and high cholesterol. His elevated blood sugar, LDL (bad cholesterol), and triglycerides (blood fat formed from carbohydrates) didn't help. To top it off, his low HDL (good cholesterol) contributed to the clogged arteries.

He could only walk a short distance without chest pains (angina), and he often needed to sit down to rest or sometimes even take nitroglycerin. This had added to his weight problems.

At this point, he was ready to do anything. I gave him a plan to help reverse his condition.

By following the 7 Systems Plan, he made tremendous gains. His vessel condition improved immensely, and he lost 40 pounds. He ate real food, took key nutrients, and fixed his Delivery System. Most of all, he began enjoying life rather than living in fear. The following year, he went to Colorado to hunt elk with his grandson. He spent the week hiking through the mountains and having a great time.

Sometime later, Ray's cardiologist wanted an angiogram because of the seriousness of the first test. This second angiogram showed that the coronary vessels had opened up again. He told me that his doctors thought there must have been a mistake on the first image because this change was impossible. Back in 1990, when this test was performed, reversing vessel damage in the heart was unheard of. However, Ray went on to live another 28 years because he followed the steps that you're reading about in this book.

If you can get your Delivery System working for you, you too can experience a more enjoyable life. Your body can heal itself if you give it what it needs. If you need proof, look at any of my patients who have done this. By following the 7 Systems Plan, they have begun to open blocked arteries and stopped using insulin, statins, and diabetic medication—within weeks, not months. Always work with your doctor when changing any medications you are currently on.

Although this plan takes effort, the increase in quality of life is unbelievable.

Why Your Delivery System Is Working Against You

Your transformation story can be just as powerful as Ray's. His problems were preventable and, in many ways, reversible.

Anybody can damage their Delivery System by eating the wrong foods and ignoring crucial nutrients. Sugar and bad fats "scratch" the lining of your blood vessels. If your LDL cholesterol is too high, it leaves deposits in these damaged areas, causing plaque or blockage.

Some nutrients are called *essential nutrients because* your body cannot produce them and it cannot function correctly without them. You need to deliver these essential nutrients to your cells regularly (preferably daily). When there is a breakdown in delivery (intake), the cells and your overall health suffer. Obesity, heart disease, stroke, diabetes, and many other diseases have their origin in a breakdown of the Delivery System.

The consequences of dysfunction in this System are severe. Fatty streaks in blood vessels at age 10 become plaque at age 20. This can trigger a heart attack at age 40. Diabetes progresses even faster than other diseases. Remember the term "adult onset diabetes"? We had to get rid of this name for type 2 diabetes because now children are developing this disease.

If you're over the age of 10, chances are that you either have these problems or will have them soon. They will either kill you or make your life miserable. Thankfully, there is another option. Fixing this System will tip the scales in your favor.

Since this System is complicated, we'll break it down into pieces to explain how it works. You cannot fix this System without first understanding the nutrients themselves and how they are delivered. Let's get started.

Why Fats Are Working Against You

Here's a quick rundown on fats and how they are delivered.

Dietary fat provides your body with essential fatty acids that it cannot produce by itself. These particular fats are used for

- Brain development and function
- Controlling inflammation
- Blood clotting
- Hormone production (adrenal hormones, estrogen, androgen, progesterone)
- Energy
- Transportation of essential nutrients
- Cell repair, fighting infection, and building bone density
- The thermal layer that helps keep us warm
- And much more

Fats cannot travel the "streets" of your body without a delivery vehicle. I like to call these vehicles "taxis." The liver produces taxis called LDL and VLDL cholesterol. They pick up the fats you eat from the Digestive System and deliver them to cells throughout your body. After delivery, these taxis return to the liver to park. The whole delivery process takes about 12 hours, and peak traffic occurs about three hours after eating.

Too much of the wrong food or problems with the taxis can cause traffic jams that start a chain reaction of accidents. These accidents can damage your blood vessels (causing fatty streaks).

Ever feel sluggish after a large, bad meal? Most Americans eat too many bad fats and bad carbohydrates. If you eat a single fast food meal, the traffic in your blood vessels can be reduced by 25% for hours.[6] You're depriving your muscles, organs, and tissues of nutrients that they need to function correctly.

If there are too many taxis on your body's streets (LDL, VLDL, and triglycerides), it's difficult for anything to get where it needs to go. It is vital that you consume appropriate amounts of the right fats and carbohydrates to keep your Delivery System functioning properly.

Once the fats have been delivered, your body has to move used up, unwanted material (cholesterol) out of your body. For this job, your liver uses the delivery vehicle HDL. It acts like a garbage truck going throughout the vessels, picking up cholesterol and returning it to the liver for disposal.

Problems with this part of the Delivery System lead to vessel disease. See the lab tests at the end of the chapter or 7SystemsPlan.com for lab resources, an easy way to understand them, and helpful tools to determine your risk level.

There is a lot you may not know about fat.
Look up any article or tune in to any health program, and you will get an abundance of information and "expert" opinions on our most hated three-letter word—*fat*.

Most people don't want to talk about fat because it is a sore subject. We have been programmed to hate it on our bodies and secretly love it in our food. Messages like "just add more butter!" and "eat low-fat or else!" add to the confusion.

The 7 Systems Plan makes sense of all this confusion and explains exactly what your body does with fat. The truth is that you actually need fat—the healthy types of fat, that is.

If you want to lose weight, avoid heart disease and cancer, prevent Alzheimer's disease, and live a healthy life, you must understand fats. Some fats can kill you, and some can save your life. The balance and quantity of fats are two important keys.

A Word of Caution About Choosing a Low-Fat Diet:

Remember, sugar and fats are added to food to make it taste good. Going on a low-fat diet often means settling for one high in sugar. A low-fat Oreo cookie may have 50 calories while a regular Oreo cookie has 53. The significance is that the cookie with the fat in it takes longer to break down and get into your bloodstream than the cookie with sugar alone.

Without fat, the sugar will shoot through your stomach and get into your bloodstream quicker. This causes your blood sugar and insulin to spike. These calories are stored as fat on your belly. If a product is low-fat and in a box or a bag, you need to take caution and look at the ingredients. Natural foods that have the right fats are always a better option.

There are different categories, or types, of fat.

Natural Fats

- Saturated
- Polyunsaturated
- Monounsaturated

All natural sources of fat include varying amounts of all three types.

Unnatural Fats

- Trans fat (also known as hydrogenated and partially hydrogenated oils)

Fats are the most calorie-dense macronutrient with nine calories per gram—that's twice as many as protein and carbohydrates. All types of fat are equally fattening.

If you've ever eaten a low-fat diet, you will have noticed two things: The food does not taste as good, and you are not as satisfied. Since fats take longer to digest than carbohydrates, they tend to keep you satisfied longer and make you less hungry. A low-fat diet can slow your metabolism down significantly (as you saw in Chapter One). It is not as simple as just counting calories.

Not eating the right fats in appropriate amounts will make it difficult to lose weight and will harm your health. Balance is the key.

How to Get Fats Working for You

Step 1: Understand the different fats.

Saturated Fat
This fat is good when it comes from the right sources and is not overconsumed. Saturated fat is comprised of carbon chains that are totally saturated with fatty acids, and it remains solid at room

temperature. Think of the fat on a steak, virgin coconut oil, and butter.

Because this fat is saturated, it does not become rancid quickly (there is no room for harmful molecules to attach to the carbon chains). It mostly comes from animal sources: meat, cheese, milk, and eggs. But it also comes from plant sources: avocados, coconut oil, and palm oil.

Saturated fat has been demonized, but it is necessary. It performs important jobs such as enhancing your immune function, decreasing heart risk factors, building stronger bones, improving liver function, making healthy lungs, improving brain function, and more.

The downside is that overconsumption of saturated fat is linked to heart disease and diabetes. When combined with bad carbohydrates, saturated fat can turn on the cholesterol-producing switch in your liver, causing your body to make more cholesterol. Saturated fat is bad only because we overconsume it and use too many unhealthy animal sources. As with all things in life, you must maintain the correct balance.

The fats in avocados and coconut oil are saturated, but they behave like monounsaturated fats in the body. As a result, they are better for you and have many health benefits. Personally, I prefer coconut oil when cooking food on the stove top since it is more stable at high temperatures.

Best sources of saturated fat:

- Coconut oil
- Avocados
- Pasture-raised, free-range, organic eggs
- Pasture-raised beef, lamb, and chicken

Polyunsaturated Fats (PUFAs): Omega-3 and Omega-6

Polyunsaturated fat's carbon chains are not totally saturated with fatty acids, so they are liquid at room temperature and in the refrigerator. Also, because it is not saturated, water, light, heat, and microbes can damage the fat and make it go rancid. Rancid fat not only tastes and smells bad but also hurts your body. Keeping it in a cool dark place can lengthen its shelf life. Let's look at two types of PUFAs: omega-3 and omega-6.

Omega-3:
One of the best and most important PUFAs is omega-3. Omega-3 fat is good for you and hard to overconsume. There are now over 20,000 published scientific papers that support the health benefits of omega-3. Some of these benefits include support for cardiovascular health, healthy brain development, healthy immune response, lower inflammation, and improved overall health.

One of the best sources of omega-3 is wild-caught fish. Try to eat fish twice per week. Make sure you pick from the list in Appendix A, Part One or at 7SystemsPlan.com. Focus on fish that are high in omega-3 and low in mercury. People who eat fish that is baked or broiled—not fried—have bigger brains and five times less incidence of Alzheimer's disease than average.[7]

There is no doubt that good fats make your brain work better. Dr. Lawrence Whalley reported, "People who eat oily fish or take fish oil supplements score 13 percent higher on IQ tests and are less likely to show sign of Alzheimer's disease. The results suggest that fish oil users have younger brains than non-users. The aging of the brain is being slowed down by a year or two."[8]

Omega-3 has two main families: EPA (eicosapentaenoic acid) and DHA (docosahexaenoic acid). Each performs different functions in your body. Both are essential fatty acids that your body cannot produce; therefore, you should regularly consume them.

Over the last century, there has been an 80% decline in our omega-3 intake. The average American takes in only 120 milligrams of omega-3 per day. That number should be at least 2,000 milligrams. To make matters worse, there has been a tremendous increase in the consumption of inflammatory omega-6. Refined vegetable oils (omega-6) are used in fast foods, most snack foods, cookies, crackers, processed food, and junk food.

Years ago, cows ate grass and produced meat that was high in omega-3. Now cows eat grains high in omega-6, so meat has little omega-3. Similar to people, animals become what they eat. If you feed a chicken omega-3-rich flaxseed, or if they are free-range, you get eggs high in omega-3. Some eggs have up to 600 milligrams of omega-3 per egg, but corn-fed chickens produce eggs with little omega-3.

Best sources of omega-3:

- High-omega-3, low-mercury fish
- Omega-3 (EPA/DHA) supplements (Note: 98% of omega-3 supplements are worthless; use only triglyceride forms.)
- Chia and flax seeds
- Walnuts
- Kiwifruit
- Black raspberries

Omega-6:
Omega-6 fat can be good for you, but you really need very little of it, and it must come from the right sources. If overconsumed, it sets up an inflammatory cascade that leads to cancer, heart disease, arthritis, and most chronic diseases. In his book *Toxic Fats*, Barry Sears says that the underlying cause of most chronic disease is inflammation caused by an imbalance of fats.

Omega-6 comes mostly from seeds, grain, seed oils (like corn, soy, safflower, and sunflower oil), and meat that is grain fed. It is also an essential fatty acid and, like omega-3, it has several families. Some of the families are helpful while others are harmful.

Best sources of omega-6:

- Nuts
- Seeds
- Borage or evening primrose oil

With PUFAs, it is all about balance. Fatty acids from fat make up part of our cell membranes and blood vessels (including brain cells, muscle cells, and nerve cells). The fat we eat is incorporated into our cell membranes.

A fluid cell membrane is critical for healthy cells and a healthy Delivery System. Some fats are more fluid and produce a cell membrane with better function, allowing good nutrients and hormones into the cell more efficiently. Omega-3 DHA is an essential fatty acid providing optimal fluidity to the cell membrane.

Consuming the wrong fats can result in poorly functioning cell membranes. Vegetable and grain oils high in omega-6, saturated fat (animal fat), and hydrogenated oils make a membrane that is more plastic than fluid. This will not let in the nutrients and hormones that the cell needs.

If the cells lining your blood vessels are high in omega-3, the platelets (blood clot cells) bounce along freely and don't get stuck on the vessel wall. This keeps the cells in your bloodstream from clumping and forming plaque.

If your vessels are high in omega-6, there is a greater chance of clots and plaque formation. These are the first signs of heart and arterial disease. The average American diet is high in omega-6, trans fat, and saturated fat. As a result, the average American suffers from inferior cell membranes and vessel lining.

Monounsaturated Fat (MUFA): Omega-9

This fat is good for you, and you should be consuming more of it. Studies show that MUFA lowers bad cholesterol, reduces heart disease, decreases stroke, improves insulin levels, and improves blood sugar. It is a healthy fat and functions as a key part of the 7 Systems Plan.

MUFA is liquid at room temperature and solid or cloudy when you put it in the refrigerator. It is more saturated than PUFA oil and therefore does not go rancid as quickly (though it should still be kept in a cool dark place).

Olive oil is the perfect example of a MUFA. Olives and nuts also have significant amounts of omega-9. All oils, nuts, and seeds have a combination of different fats in them, so it is important to use the ones with more omega-3 and omega-9 than omega-6.

Best sources of omega-9:

- Nuts and seeds
- Olives and avocados
- Extra virgin olive, MCT, and coconut oil (for cooking)

In summary, use oils that are highest in omega-9 (e.g. olive oil) and omega-3 fat (e.g. fish oil) and lowest in saturated fat (animal fat) and omega-6 fat (e.g. vegetable oils).

For a chart on fats and oils, visit 7SystemsPlan.com.

Step 2: Villainize unnatural fats.

Trans, hydrogenated, and partially hydrogenated fats are always bad in any amount because they are polyunsaturated fat that has been artificially transformed into a more saturated form. They are used in nearly all processed foods to help preserve their shelf life. They are the absolute worst of all fats.

To prevent PUFA from going rancid, manufacturers bubble hydrogen gas through the oil so that there are no open bonds where oxygen can attach and make it go rancid. During the hydrogenation process, fat molecules are "twisted" into different shapes. These different shapes are not recognized by your body, and they cause damage—especially to your blood vessels. They also replace the good fats in your cell membranes, impairing cell function. Remember that the fat you eat (good or bad) is incorporated into your cell membranes and vessel walls.

Many people wonder, "How bad can hydrogenated fats really be?"

More than 5 grams per serving of these fats is associated with a 25% increase in ischemic heart disease. A recent study showed that one additional serving of French fries per week for children between the ages of three and five increased the adult risk of breast cancer by 27%.[9] There appears to be an increased negative effect when you combine bad fats with carbohydrates.

Fast foods are notorious for their trans fat. Up to 30% of the oil used in restaurants is can be this bad fat. If you want to make a healthy choice, avoid processed foods and eating out too often. Fortunately, some restaurants have decreased their use of trans fat, but processed foods are still loaded with it. Always read the labels, and avoid all foods with trans fat, hydrogenated oil, and partially hydrogenated oil.

They should not be in your shopping cart or your body.

Best sources of unnatural fats:

• None!

Identify Your Fat Intake

The ratio of omega-6 to omega-3 in your cells should be 2:1. Studies show that if your ratio is greater than 15:1, you are at risk for chronic disease. The average American's ratio is 20:1! You can determine your levels with a simple test. See the end of the chapter or 7SystemsPlan.com for information.

Step 3: Understand cholesterol and statin drugs.

A discussion on fat is not complete without addressing cholesterol. Although cholesterol does not contain any fatty acids, it is classified as fat because it has some of the same chemical and physical characteristics.

Although cholesterol has been demonized, it performs many important jobs in your body ranging from maintaining healthy cell membranes to building vital hormones and vitamins. This important nutrient is a part of every cell, and your body cannot function without it.

Only 10% of cholesterol in the blood comes from diet and the remaining 90% (800–1,500 mg per day) is produced in the liver. This is why—contrary to popular belief—cutting down on cholesterol in the diet has a limited benefit. It is important to know that when you eat too much saturated fat and sugar, your liver cranks up the production of cholesterol. Limiting your consumption of these two things is a key to controlling cholesterol.

The types of fats and carbohydrates you eat are a much bigger problem than the amount of cholesterol you consume. If you want to control your cholesterol, then keep your liver functioning correctly. Instead of focusing so much on dietary cholesterol, follow the 7 Systems Plan.

Patients ask me if there is a potential problem in driving cholesterol too low with cholesterol medication. I believe there is. Not having enough cholesterol can result in serious health consequences.

Fifteen million Americans are taking a statin drug to lower their cholesterol. Statins work by blocking the manufacture of cholesterol in the liver.[10] This decreases the number of "taxis," the LDL and VLDL cholesterol that can deposit fats in your vessel walls. Unfortunately, it also reduces the good HDL (the "garbage truck") that picks up cholesterol from the vessel walls and returns it to the liver.

Lower cholesterol can indicate a lower risk for heart disease, and studies show that taking a statin drug has a small benefit for people with high LDL cholesterol. However, new studies seem to indicate that the benefits of statins come more from their anti-inflammatory effect than their cholesterol-lowering effect.[11] In Chapter Six, you will learn natural, powerful ways to decrease inflammation.

Taking statins does not come without risk.[12] Up to 20% of statin users experience serious side effects including an increase in risk for diabetes, Alzheimer's disease, sexual dysfunction, and nerve and muscle pain.

Statins are known to lower the production of Coenzyme Q10 (CoQ10). This may be the cause of muscle pain that becomes permanent for some patients. This enzyme is also critical for preventing heart attacks. No one should be taking a statin drug without also being on a CoQ10 supplement.

To make matters worse, new studies show that if you take a statin drug, you are likely to forfeit any or all health benefits of exercise![13] Statins can poison the energy-producing part of your cells (mitochondria), impairing your body's ability to produce energy.

A safe and effective way to reduce your heart attack risk is to follow the 7 Systems Plan. Adding three grams of omega-3 per day to your diet improves fat transportation and lowers VLDL. Omega-3 also has a strong anti-inflammatory effect. Some studies show it to be more effective in reducing heart attack risk than statins, without any of the bad side effects.

Why Proteins Are Working Against You

Fats are the first macronutrient and proteins are the second. Your body needs proteins to make essential amino acids. These amino acids are used to

- Make enzymes, hormones, and other body chemicals
- Build and repair muscle, bone, cartilage, skin, and blood
- Serve as taxis for hormones, vitamins, minerals, lipids, and other materials
- Help your body maintain the ideal acid/alkaline balance
- Function as an important part of your immune function
- Alter inflammation, increase energy production, and help you eat less

Proteins are carried through the blood by two different taxis—amino acids and albumin—which are produced in the liver. When quality protein is not taken in and delivered to the cells, all cellular processes are impaired and you lose muscle.

Although it's important to get enough protein each day, overconsuming protein (especially animal protein) can cause many health problems:

- It stimulates pathways (IGF-1) that increase cancer risk.[14]
- It stimulates the mTOR intracellular signaling pathway (directly related to cell proliferation) that can increase

cancer risk. Valter Longo, director of the USC Longevity Institute, thinks the risks of a high-protein diet are comparable to smoking.[15]

- It increases the acid load to the kidneys, potentially damaging sensitive kidney cells.[16]
- It makes your body more acidic, which can impair the function of multiple Systems. (We will discuss this more in Chapter Seven.)

How to Get Protein Working for You

Step 1: Consume the perfect amount of protein.

Studies show that you can lose weight by increasing your protein intake. However, the source of your protein is very important. Proteins have just four calories per gram, and the energy your body uses to digest protein is significantly more than for carbohydrates or fat. Since protein takes longer to digest, it stays in your stomach longer, making you feel more satisfied. It also helps slow the movement of carbohydrates into the bloodstream, keeping your blood sugar at a good level for a longer time. Eat some protein with each of your meals and snacks. It should be the first thing you eat because you'll get full faster and feel more satisfied.

There is much controversy over the amount of protein you need per day. I believe you should always get at least 50 grams per day. If you are active and exercising, you may need 150 grams per day. It is important to note that some studies indicate that our body can only utilize about 30 grams of protein at a time. If you eat 50 grams at one time, you may not be able to use it all.[17] Spread it out throughout the day, and don't go over 30 grams per meal. Also be aware that as we age, we do need more protein to maintain our muscle.

American diets are frequently too high in animal protein. Try eating more plant protein and less meat.

How much protein do you need?

Multiply your ideal weight (not actual weight if you are overweight) by 0.72 if you are active or 0.36 if you are not active.

For example, if your ideal weight is 160lbs, here is the correct formula:

- If you are active (160 × 0.72), consume 115 grams of protein daily.
- If you are not active (160 × 0.36), consume 57 grams of protein daily.

Do this:

- Add up the grams of protein you eat each day. Find your perfect balance, and do your best to stick to it. You'll have more lean muscle mass and not lose muscle after all your efforts to build it.

Step 2: Consume the perfect proteins.

Protein from Beans (Legumes)

You need to eat more beans. They are the perfect food, packed with protein (14–16 grams per cup), good carbohydrates, and only 1 gram of fat in a cup. Among the best legumes are chickpeas, black beans, red beans, white beans, green peas, lima beans, pinto beans, and lentils. Eating a half cup per day is a great goal (unless you have blood sugar or inflammation problems, in which case you may need to limit your bean consumption). Some Digestive Systems do not handle legumes well. If you have ongoing symptoms after eating legumes, avoid them.

Protein from Eggs

Eggs contain 6–8 grams of protein each. They have been demonized over the years, but are now coming back into favor. Eggs have the highest quality protein of almost any food. Eggs contain good fats, many vitamins, and key minerals. They are also rich in amino acids and antioxidants that support brain function. Eggs are one of only three foods that contain any significant amounts of vitamin D, and they have been shown to boost HDL (good cholesterol).

Dietary cholesterol does not translate into high levels of blood cholesterol. Studies reveal that high-egg diets have no effect on cholesterol levels, even at 12 eggs per week.[18]

If you are going to eat eggs, choose organic, pasture-raised, or free-range.

- Organic means that the chickens are fed organic food, which is much better than the alternative.
- Pasture-raised or free-range means the chickens are allowed to roam free rather than spend their lives in a cage.
- The absolute best eggs come from a farmer who lets his chickens run free and feeds them organic feeds.

Protein from Nuts and Seeds

These have 4–8 grams of protein per quarter cup. They are a great source of both protein and good fats. A recent 30-year study showed that people who ate a small handful of nuts per day had a 20% decrease in mortality from all causes.[19]

Many studies show that nuts can help you lose weight. In a study comparing people who ate a low-calorie diet with complex carbohydrates and people who ate a low-calorie diet with almonds, the nut group had a 50% greater decrease in their weight, waist circumference, and body fat percentage.[20] Nuts are clearly a better snack than whole grains.

Another study from the *Journal of Obesity* shows that eating nuts two or more times per week helped keep people from gaining weight (compared with people who do not eat nuts).[21] As a general practice, eating nuts will help you keep weight off more successfully.

Eat Nuts, Lose Weight

Since nuts are high in fat, eating them should make you gain weight, but studies prove the opposite. There are four reasons why:

- Nuts are hard to digest, and up to 70% of their calories can be lost in digestion.
- Nuts satisfy you, so you feel full and eat less food throughout the day.
- Nuts boost metabolism and burn up more of your own fat.
- Up to 10% of the calories from nuts are lost in feces.

Weight loss is not the only benefit of eating nuts. People who eat nuts have lower blood pressure and higher HDL (good cholesterol). They are less likely to be obese or have metabolic syndrome, high blood sugar, or heart disease.

Among the best nuts are walnuts, almonds, Brazil nuts, macadamias, pecans, and pistachios. Peanuts are the least healthy choice. While raw nuts have more health benefits, you may not enjoy them as much. If you can eat them raw, do so. Otherwise, eat them roasted—but pay attention to the oils used in processing.

Do this:

- Eat more beans, eggs, nuts, and seeds.

Step 3: Make healthy meat choices.

Americans eat 222 pounds of meat per person per year, more than any other country on the planet! You do not need to become a vegetarian, but you do need to decrease the amount you eat and change the quality of the meat in your diet. If you're eating a steak, get a 3-ounce serving, not a 9-ounce.

Eating less meat is not that hard if you follow the 7 Systems Plan. My patients eat more plant protein and limited amounts of fish that is low in mercury and high in omega-3 as well as pasture-raised beef, poultry, and lamb when possible.

You might wonder how you will get enough protein if you cut down your meat intake. One common misconception is that vegetables have no protein, or animal protein is superior to plant protein.

Consider this: 100 calories of broccoli have 7 grams of protein. Eating a 10-ounce box of frozen spinach gives you 10 grams of protein.

Do this:

- Decrease your meat consumption and increase plant protein.
- Make good meat choices.

Why Carbohydrates Are Working Against You

The body has two main fuel sources: carbohydrates and stored fat. Like proteins, carbohydrates have four calories per gram. Carbohydrates are your body's preferred fuel source; that is their sole function. Your body breaks carbohydrates down into glucose, which can be stored as energy or fat. Glucose can move through the bloodstream without a taxi.

Unlike the other macronutrients—fat and protein—carbohydrates are not essential. They are only used for energy. Most people eat too many of the wrong carbohydrates. Eating bad carbohydrates in excess causes many of the diseases plaguing people today.

Bad carbohydrates cause weight gain and block your body from burning fat. You can store about 1,500 calories of carbohydrates as glycogen in your liver and muscles for later use. Any excess will be stored as fat. If you limit the number of calories and bad carbohydrates you eat every day, your body will be forced to use up this glycogen and then burn stored fat. Following the 7 Systems Plan will make this happen.

High glucose levels in the blood (from carbohydrates) create problems. Excess glucose is converted into triglycerides (a blood fat) and eventually gets stored in fat cells. Triglycerides are an important measure of heart health and can indicate carbohydrate addiction. If your levels are greater than 200, then you're most likely a carbohydrate addict and may be moving toward diabetes. You can lower your triglycerides quickly by decreasing your bad carbohydrate intake.

Although glucose does not need a taxi to be delivered, it does need help getting into the cells. For glucose to enter most cells, it needs the hormone insulin. Overconsumption of sugar makes the cells resistant to insulin, so it can't do its job. Problems with this part of the Delivery System lead to weight gain, diabetes, dementia, and many other problems.

We will talk more about this in Chapter Five, but for now, see the lab section at the end of the chapter or 7SystemsPlan. com for tests to determine your risk for blood sugar problems caused by excess carbohydrate consumption.

How to Get Carbohydrates Working for You

Step 1: Consume good carbohydrates.

If you eat junk food, you can surpass the recommended amount of carbohydrates your body needs in one meal very easily. But it's almost impossible to consume too many carbohydrates *if* they come in the form of vegetables. The 7 Systems Plan suggests using vegetables as the cornerstone of your diet. Vegetables are low in calories, high in fiber, and packed with all the vitamins and minerals you need. A wonderful side benefit is that they fill you up fast.

There are many ways to eat vegetables: raw, steamed, cooked, sautéed, juiced, or even sprouted or fermented. Good carbohydrates will make you smarter and better looking. They will improve your mental well-being too.

> Sprouts have about 30 times the nutrient value of the vegetables they turn into. Since they are power-packed with nutrients, you should consume them regularly. Some of my favorite sprouts are alfalfa, broccoli, and radish.

Simple vs. Complex Carbohydrates
A carb is a carb, right? Wrong. Think about sitting down to eat 22 cups of broccoli today. You would eat about 112 grams of carbohydrates and 600 calories. The task would be difficult. But the same number of carbohydrates and calories are in four cans of soft drinks. Drinking four cans wouldn't be too difficult for most people.

Although they contain the same number of carbohydrates and calories, the fat you would store from each would not be the same. The kind of calories you consume greatly influences obesity. It's not just the calories or even the carbohydrates you consume but the *composition* of the carbohydrates that matter.

Carbohydrates break down into sugars and come in many forms, but we are going to focus on two: disaccharides (simple or short chains of sugar molecules) and polysaccharides (complex or long chains of sugar molecules).

Think of sugar molecules like beads on two necklaces: one has a few beads and one has many.

A simple chain with one or two beads would be easily broken down in your Digestive System—therefore, sugar enters your bloodstream quickly. The more rapidly it enters the bloodstream, the more damage it does to your body and the more weight you gain.

A Few of The 127 Names for Sugar

- Brown sugar
- Corn sweetener
- Corn syrup
- Fructose
- Fruit juice concentrate
- Glucose
- High fructose corn syrup
- Honey
- Invert sugar
- Lactose
- Maltose
- Molasses
- Raw sugar
- Sucrose (table sugar)

Sugar substitutes include

- Acesulfame K (Sunett)
- Aspartame (NutraSweet, Equal)
- Erythritol
- Mannitol
- Saccharin
- Sorbitol
- Stevia
- Sucralose (Splenda)
- Xylitol

The longer strings of beads are complex sugar molecules. They take longer to break down and enter the bloodstream. The slower they enter, the longer it takes for you to feel hungry and the more your body benefits.

To sum it up: Eating too much sugar or too many simple carbohydrates pushes your body to store the calories as fat and increases your hunger and your waistline.

Sugar
For the majority of people, carbohydrates make up 50% or more of their daily diet. Sugar and flour are their two biggest calorie sources. Sugar consumption is now at 152 pounds per year per person, up from 40 pounds in 1980. There are now 600,000 food products available, and 80% of these products contain added sugar.

8–15% of calories in the average American diet come from soft drinks alone. Here are a couple of facts about people who consume soft drinks:

- Kids who drink 1 can per day increase their risk of obesity by 60%.
- Women who drink 1 can per day increase their risk of type 2 diabetes and cardiovascular disease by 80%.

On average, children consume 34 teaspoons of sugar per day. Consuming more than 8 teaspoons per day diminishes their chances of achieving a healthy life.

There should be about 5 grams of sugar (one teaspoon) in every person's blood at any given time. There can be 20 grams of glucose in half a candy bar, which would quadruple your blood sugar in 15 minutes. A 60-ounce soft drink can have up to 40 teaspoons of sugar—that's 40 times the amount your entire bloodstream should contain!

When trying to identify sugar on labels, look for "ose" at the end of the word. Many sugars end in ose, but not all of them. You must be familiar with the different names for sugar so you can pick them out when you read labels.

One of the most common types of sugar used today is fructose.

As we just discovered, when glucose enters the bloodstream it can be stored or used for energy, but the same is not true for fructose. Fructose must first pass through the liver to be metabolized. Because we overconsume fructose, it "backs up" in the liver and results in fatty liver disease, insulin resistance, and obesity. Because of its harmful effect on the liver, fructose may well be 20 times more fattening than glucose!

An example of the dangers of fructose is the Chinese diet.[22] In the 1990s (as documented in the INTERMAP study), the Chinese diet was extremely high in white rice but low in sugar. Although rice has quite a bit of glucose, it has almost no fructose. At that time, China had very little obesity and diabetes. But as the Chinese people adopted the Western diet and added sugar (glucose and fructose), they created a recipe for disaster, and now the prevalence of diabetes in China is greater than in the U.S.

Sources of fructose include sugar, honey, fruit, and high fructose corn syrup (HFCS). Since table sugar (sucrose) is half glucose and half fructose, it is especially dangerous. Although fruit contains fructose, reasonable amounts do not seem to be a problem (however, fruit juices contain astronomically high sugar concentrations). HFCS is the primary source of calories in most diets and the worst of all sugars, damaging both your weight and health. Studies show that our country's weight gain since 1976 has very closely paralleled our increased use of HFCS.[23]

Part of maintaining a healthy lifestyle is identifying hidden sugars. Many of us unknowingly dump huge amounts of sugar into our bodies.

- A low-fat yogurt can have the same sugar content as a soft drink.

- A serving of tomato sauce can do the same thing to your blood sugar as two Oreo cookies.
- The sugar content of a glass of orange juice equals that of a soft drink.

There are some sugar substitutes and sugar alcohols (ending in "ol") that are better options than sugar. My favorites would be stevia, Truvia, erythritol and xylitol. Bad sugar substitutes are not an option. Besides destroying your good gut bacteria, recent reports reveal the risk of stroke in those consuming one or more artificially-sweetened sodas per day was almost tripled, with a similar finding for Alzheimer's risk.[24]

Step 2: Use the glycemic index.

A food's glycemic index (GI) indicates the speed at which its carbohydrates are delivered to your bloodstream and raise your blood sugar. High-GI foods are some of the biggest contributors to obesity today. Many studies also connect them to diabetes and heart disease. Without maintaining a low-GI diet, you will not be able to maintain health and a good weight.

Low Glycemic Index: < 55
- Dried peas and beans (legumes)
- Barley and bulgur (cracked wheat)
- Most vegetables and fruits
- Nuts and seeds
- Most dairy products

Medium Glycemic Index: 56–69
- Most root vegetables
- Most whole grains (e.g. brown rice, rolled oats)

High Glycemic Index: > 70
- Desserts
- Refined grains (e.g. instant oatmeal)

- Soft drinks
- Sweetened sports drinks

Eating high-GI meals can cause serious problems. One bad meal tends to set you up to eat another and another. When overweight kids eat a high-GI first meal, they eat 81% more at their next meal.[25] Eating a healthy, well-balanced, low-GI first meal of the day is imperative if you want to lose weight.

Now you know that the faster a food gets into your bloodstream, the quicker your blood sugar rises. But speed isn't all that matters. The quantity of carbohydrate in a food (its glycemic load) also affects blood sugar levels and insulin response. You need to look at a food's glycemic index *and* its glycemic load. You can access a glycemic chart at 7SystemsPlan.com.

> Although watermelon is a high-GI food, it doesn't have a high glycemic load because it is mostly water. Therefore, it's considered a high-GI food that is not too bad. A baked potato is much worse because it has a high glycemic index and a high glycemic load.

Step 3: Discover the truth about flour and grains.

If sugar were our only problem, we could deal with it. Unfortunately, it's not. On average we consume 146 pounds of flour per year. The glycemic index of sugar and flour are about the same, and they both cause significant damage.

- Two slices of bread can be the same as 2–3 teaspoons of sugar.
- One big plate of spaghetti can do the same thing to your blood sugar as eating four candy bars.

Do not be fooled by whole grain cereals. They can contain 22 grams of sugar—5 teaspoons—in just ¾ of a cup. The sugars come from sources like corn, cornmeal, brown sugar, corn flour, and corn syrup. Many cereals have six or more kinds of added sugar.[26]

Carb-Rich Foods are as Risky as Cigarettes

According to Dr. Joseph Mercola, "research suggests refined non-vegetable fiber carbs such as potatoes, bagels and breakfast cereal are as risky as smoking, increasing your risk for lung cancer by as much as 49 percent."[26]

Eating too many carbohydrates or the wrong ones can lead to obesity, diabetes, heart disease, and many other common killers. At the current rate, one in three children will develop diabetes. The good news is that since 91% of all diabetes is attributed to lifestyle, the majority of people can decrease their risk by adopting the 7 Systems Plan.

Choose good carbohydrates like vegetables, legumes (beans), and fruits. Think *pounds* of vegetables, not ounces. After a short time, you will learn to love them and—more importantly—what they do to you and how they make you feel.

Why Vitamins and Minerals Are Working Against You

Now that we have covered the macronutrients, we can discuss the micronutrients: vitamins and minerals. The daily food choices you make are the most important factor in your health, but vitamins are also a powerful tool to help you reach your potential. There are dozens of nutrients that are essential for the health of your body's most basic processes:

- Metabolism
- Energy production
- Cell division and function
- Maintenance and function of the brain, heart, immune function, lungs, skin, bone, muscle, etc.

- Growth and development
- Physical and mental well-being

Some vitamins and minerals have their own taxis. The water-soluble vitamins have proteins to carry them and the fat-soluble vitamins A, D, E, and K have to be carried by lipoproteins.

Problems in the Delivery System lead to anemia, osteoporosis, and a breakdown of all the other Systems. Most people have long-term nutritional deficiencies that promote the development of cancer, brain deterioration, and heart disease. Subtle vitamin deficiencies can also have a negative impact on immunity and overall health. As many as 8 of the top 10 causes of death are directly related to poor nutrition and these deficiencies.

Modern food is too weak to replenish our bodies' depleted cells. Because of soil depletion over the last few decades, many fruits and vegetables have lost over half their vitamins and minerals. Studies show that two peaches would have supplied the recommended daily allowance of vitamin A for an adult in 1951. Today, we would have to eat almost 53 peaches to get our daily requirement. Over the last 50 years, potatoes have lost 50% of their vitamin A, C, and D, and 20% of their calcium.

If you want to be free from debilitating disease, live a long and healthy life, and be strong, you must take nutritional supplements. Taking a daily vitamin is a simple way to prevent these deficiencies.

Unfortunately, many vitamin brands are worthless. When shopping for vitamins, only buy brands that are GMP (good manufacturing practice) certified. This is the gold standard for certification. Here are three reasons to use only certified brands:

1. *Label Claims:* When put to the test, many brands do not meet label claims. In fact, some inexpensive brands have almost nothing in them.
2. *Material Testing:* Some companies do not test the raw material they use to make supplements for contamination.

Some poor-quality supplements contain heavy metals like mercury and pesticides and chemicals like DDT and PCB. Some herbs may be adulterated with pharmaceutical drugs or toxic minerals such as lead.

Companies that carry high-quality supplements have rigorous testing procedures to ensure that no contaminants are in the product. In a 12-month period, one supplement company rejected 106 raw materials that failed to meet their quality specifications. Those raw materials were returned and probably sold to other companies that do not test their raw materials.

3. *Body Breakdown:* Make sure the supplements you take are high quality so your body can break them down during digestion. Many companies have not taken the necessary care to assess the bioavailability of their products. In one study, supplements were checked to see if they would break down fast enough to be used by a human body. 11 of the 21 tablets did not break down in time to be absorbed, and samples of 6 products did not disintegrate within one hour.[27]

It is worth spending a little more to get a good-quality supplement that is GMP certified.

How To Get Micronutrients Working For You: The Fab Five

Take only GMP certified supplements and use the five most important so that your Systems can thrive. The supplements are listed in order of priority. If you can only take one nutrient, start with number one. If you can take more, keep going down the list. Ideally, you will take all five on the list.

1. Functional Foods

The reason I have made functional food the most important on my list is that they supply many vitamins, minerals, and key nutrients. It's also a complete meal replacement—providing all the necessary macronutrients—and can meet many of your body's needs.

If you want to lose weight and support your Systems, add a functional food or product. In a randomized intervention trial of patients who had the problems described in this chapter, all the patients were put on the same good diet, but half of them added a functional food. After 12 weeks, the group taking the functional food had a significantly greater improvement in cholesterol, triglycerides, LDL, and all other lab numbers. Additionally, about 50% more patients on the functional food no longer met criteria for metabolic syndrome (prediabetes) compared with patients not taking the functional food.[28]

Having worked with weight-loss patients for over 35 years, I have found that functional foods work long-term. On the other hand, food replacement plans do not. Most people who go on food replacement programs (where they buy their meals from a company) may lose weight, but they tend to gain it all back when they stop buying the meals.

For the last 16 years, I have personally been using a functional food almost every day, as have many of my patients. Functional foods contain a specific combination of whole food macronutrient derivatives, micronutrients, and botanical extracts designed with specific therapeutic goals in mind. I use them in my office to help people lose weight, maintain an ideal body composition, lower cholesterol, reverse arterial damage, and diabetes, and support their Systems.

Functional foods contain a high-quality plant protein to help improve body composition by promoting the development of muscle mass. They also have phytonutrients (protective nutrients) from fruits and vegetables to help reverse arterial disease and significantly lower cholesterol.

If you have a specific System that is causing your weight and health problems, use the appropriate functional food or supplement as a meal replacement to help you get to your health goals. Visit 7SystemsPlan.com to see the functional foods and supplements I personally use. I also have more information in

Appendix A Part Five and provide a simple way to order these foods for yourself through my online store.

2. Multivitamin with Phytonutrients
I like to call this supplement the "magic pill." It has been shown to reduce chronic disease, improve mood and immune function, decrease infection, improve intelligence scores in children, decrease inflammation, and much more.

My rules for taking a multivitamin are that it must be GMP certified and natural (no synthetics). It must also contain the right forms of vitamins (some forms are not as usable by your body as others), and it should include phytonutrients.

My favorite multivitamin is called Essential Multi. It contains micronutrients that recharge your cellular health and nourish cells. It also provides phytonutrients and essential vitamins and minerals that your body needs to support its proper function.

Essential Multi is a comprehensive multivitamin and mineral formula with patented ingredients vital for optimal health and longevity. Some of them you may have heard of like lutein, lycopene, and resveratrol. It features vitamins your body can use immediately as well as other essential vitamins and minerals for cellular and targeted body support that will aid your brain, eyes, vision, heart, immune function, mitochondria, liver, and metabolism.

3. Vitamin D3
Over the last 10 years, vitamin D3 has been moving up my priority list so that it is now #3. More and more studies reveal its importance. It's a critical vitamin for maintaining proper health because it influences about 3,000 of your 30,000 genes and helps prevent a multitude of diseases—from heart disease to the common cold.

It is impossible to acquire adequate vitamin D from your diet alone, but your body can produce it with enough sun exposure. Vitamin D is produced when your skin is exposed to UV-B radiation from the sun. To get enough vitamin D, your body needs 15–20 minutes of full body exposure to sunlight per day.

Obviously, in the northern latitudes, this is not possible. In Los Angeles, your body can produce vitamin D year-round, but in Denver, vitamin D production ceases from October to March. The farther north you go, the more difficult it is to produce your own vitamin D.

Latitude is not the only problem. If you use sunblock, you decrease your vitamin D production by up to 95%. Also, dark skin makes it harder to produce vitamin D, and being overweight makes storing vitamin D more difficult.

Here are some facts about vitamin D:

- Low vitamin D contributes to weight gain. People with the highest body mass indexes (BMIs) are the most likely to be vitamin D deficient, and overweight people have better success at losing weight when they increase their vitamin D levels.
- A study of more than 4,600 women age 65 and older showed that having low vitamin D levels can contribute to mild weight gain.[30]
- In another study, more than 80% of obese adolescents seeking weight-loss surgery were found to be deficient in vitamin D.[31] A significant number had severe deficiencies, and teens with the highest BMIs were the most likely to be vitamin D deficient.
- Low vitamin D can cause chronic musculoskeletal pain.
- Vitamin D reduces cancer risk by up to 67% when blood levels are 40 ng/ml compared to less than 20.[32]
- Your heart attack risk is twice as high if your vitamin D levels are less than 34.[33]
- Vitamin D has been used to lower blood pressure in patients.[34]
- Vitamin D has been shown to decrease blood sugar problems by improving insulin sensitivity.[35]

- Multiple sclerosis is associated with vitamin D deficiency, as are other autoimmune diseases.
- It can reduce the chances of getting influenza up to 77%.
- Vitamin D decreases inflammation, the cause of many degenerative diseases. It seems to act as a brake on overactive immune function, inhibiting inflammatory cytokines.
- Sex and orgasm intensity increase when your blood vitamin D is at a good level.

We now know there are two forms of vitamin D. As doctors learn more about the importance of vitamin D, they are prescribing it more often. Unfortunately, many of them are using D2. Ergocalciferol (D2) is not normally found in humans. It's potentially toxic and may not raise your blood D levels. Since this supplement may increase your risk of death by 2% according to some studies, do *not* take it.[36]

Cholecalciferol (D3) is the vitamin you want. In my clinic, I have found that for many patients it takes about 5,000 IU per day to keep them at a safe level (above 50 ng/ml in the blood). It can take a much higher dose than that to get you to a safe level, and this may take months. High levels of vitamin D should not be taken without lab tests and a doctor's supervision as too much D can be toxic. Have your test done today to determine your vitamin D needs. Request a 25(OH)D blood test.[37]

4. Omega-3 EPA/DHA

Omega-3 is an essential fatty acid. Since your body can't produce it naturally, you must consume it. Omega-3 comes with some amazing benefits, including a decrease in fatal arrhythmias, cancer, and Alzheimer's. It also corrects skin problems, dilates arteries, decreases inflammation, and boosts immune function.

Here are some facts about omega-3:

- Having the ideal omega-3 balance has been shown, in some studies, to reduce the risk of primary heart attack by up to 90%.[27]

- In animal studies, fish oil caused weight loss and also appeared to stop animals from gaining weight, even when they were given free access to food. In the same studies, it was shown to reduce the number of fat cells, especially in the abdominal area.
- Omega-3 significantly decreases the risk of Alzheimer's disease and helps slow down brain aging. Just eating fish once a week can reduce your risk of developing Alzheimer's disease by up to 60%.[38]

After checking your vitamin D levels, the BrainSpan test discussed at the end of this chapter should be second on your priority list. Another way to find out if you're deficient in omega-3 is simply to rub the back of your arm. If you have dry skin or little bumps on the back of your arm, you may be low in omega-3.

I recommended to my patients that they take 2,000–5,000 mg per day of an omega-3 supplement containing both EPA and DHA.

5. Probiotics

To keep your Digestive System working correctly, you need probiotics—the good bacteria that coat the inside and outside of your body.

It's estimated that you have 10 times more bacteria than the number of cells in your body. This means 100,000 bacteria/ml of fluid in your stomach and 1 trillion in every ml of stool in your bowel. There are 400 different types of bacteria in your gut alone! Overall, you have about three pounds of bacteria in and on your body.

Don't get anxious. You need these friends.

Here are some facts about probiotics:

- More than 200 studies show that probiotics may relieve 170+ diseases.
- Probiotics have been found to influence the activity of hundreds of your genes, helping them to express in a positive, health-promoting manner.

- Type 2 diabetes in humans is associated with compositional changes in intestinal microbiota.
- Microbial imbalances are associated with gastritis, irritable bowel syndrome, inflammatory bowel disease, food allergies, ulcers, and yeast infections. Good bacteria can help your Digestive System function well, reduce constipation, decrease urogenital infections, and even improve the digestion of milk.
- Probiotics improve your immune function.
- The association between arthritis and intestinal inflammation has been established in many studies. Skin problems and autoimmune diseases can also be triggered by this inflammation. Good bacteria help silence these issues.
- The bacteria found in the Digestive Systems of lean people and obese people are radically different.

Many people think that they do not need to take probiotics because they eat yogurt. Unfortunately, many yogurts do not contain any significant amounts of beneficial bacteria. You may have to eat 74 tubs of certain types of yogurt to get the good bacteria found in just one probiotic capsule.

If you consume soft drinks, use artificial sweeteners, eat meat from the store, or drink chlorinated water, you could be killing off the beneficial bacteria in your intestinal tract. It is imperative that you replace these bacteria regularly. I suggest that you take at least two probiotic capsules per week on an empty stomach. If you have digestive problems or have been on antibiotic therapy, you should take one capsule per day on an empty stomach to get your beneficial bacteria back up to an adequate level.

In humans, probiotic use is linked to healthy weight loss. People with weight problems should use a supplement called UltraBiotic Integrity.

When taking a probiotic, make sure your supplement is GMP certified and contains the most helpful bacteria. At 7SystemsPlan.com, I provide a list of probiotics that can survive stomach acid. These particular probiotics have the potency to give your body what it needs.

Quick Recap:

Fat

- Some fats are essential. You must get enough of the right types on a daily basis.
- Saturated fat is necessary and comes mostly from animal sources and a few plants. Overconsuming animal protein makes it easy to take in too much saturated fat. Plant fat is preferable to animal fat.
- Polyunsaturated fat (PUFA) can be omega-3 or omega-6, and both are essential. Most people do not consume enough omega-3 and eat way too much omega-6. You should maintain a 2:1 (omega-6 to omega-3) ratio in your diet and cells.
- Grass-fed meat, some fish, and free-range eggs are high in omega-3. Most conventionally raised meats, eggs, and grain oils are high in omega-6.
- Monounsaturated fat (MUFA) has many health benefits and should be consumed often.
- Olive and coconut oil are two of the best oils to use. Nuts, olives, and flaxseed are good sources of MUFA.
- Trans fats, partially hydrogenated and hydrogenated fats, are bad in any amount. Consuming these fats results in many negative consequences.
- Decreasing your processed food intake will help you achieve your health goals.
- Cholesterol is an important nutrient.
- Following the 7 Systems Plan will fix cholesterol problems without the use of harmful drugs.

Protein

- Eating the best kinds and the right amount of protein is important for your health.

- Calculate your protein requirements and make sure you get the right amount.
- Beans, nuts, eggs, and vegetables are all good protein sources. Plant protein is even better for you than animal protein.

Carbohydrates

- Overconsumption of bad carbohydrates is the root of obesity, heart disease, stroke, and diabetes.
- The simpler a carbohydrate is, the quicker it enters the bloodstream and the more damage it does.
- Most people consume too much sugar and seriously underconsume vegetables.
- A food's glycemic index indicates the speed at which its carbohydrates are delivered to your bloodstream and raise your blood sugar.
- Low-GI foods should make up the majority of your diet.
- Medium-GI foods should be a smaller part of your diet.
- High-GI foods should be a rare treat.

Vitamins and Minerals

- Use only GMP certified supplements.
- Consider using a functional food as your first meal each day. Use one that will help support your weakest System.
- Take a multivitamin each day.
- Have your vitamin D level checked, and keep it to 70 ng/mL. Many people require 5,000 IU per day to stay in the safe zone.
- Have your omega-3 level checked, and take at least 2 grams of EPA/DHA omega-3 per day.
- Take probiotics daily for a month to get your microbiome (gut bacteria) healthy, and then take at least two per week on an empty stomach.

Proven Steps to Fix Your Delivery System:

(Check these off as you complete them. Join our free 7 Systems Plan Community for additional support and encouragement: 7SystemsPlan.com.)

☐ Eat a healthy amount of good fats daily, and avoid bad fats.

☐ Eat a healthy amount of quality protein. Move to using more plant protein and less animal protein.

☐ Avoid bad carbohydrates and load up on the good ones (often found in vegetables).

☐ Take supplements that will boost your progress.

Supplements to Support Your Delivery System

You must control your lipids and blood sugar to have a healthy Delivery System. Here is a product that I use to help patients with problems like Ray's: Dynamic Cardio-Metabolic. It offers support for healthy blood lipid profiles, a healthy insulin response, and satiation

---

Delivery System Lab Tests

Simple At-Home Test: Pulse Test

Grab a watch and check your pulse. According to studies, the higher your resting pulse, the greater your chance of dying. Ideally, your resting pulse should be about 60 beats per minute. Watch this number go down as you fix your Delivery System.

Fats

A lipid profile is a panel of several different tests used as a broad medical screening tool for abnormalities of the following lipids.

To understand your lipid profile test results, you need to look at the total values and the ratios of several different tests.

Total Cholesterol
Total cholesterol of less than 200 mg/dL is desirable, 200–239 is borderline high, and anything greater than 300 is high. The composition of this total cholesterol is of great importance, as you will learn. Total cholesterol is the sum of all "good and bad" cholesterol (HDL, LDL, and VLDL).

LDL and VLDL
These are called the bad cholesterols, but they are bad only when they are too high. They have many important functions, including regulating brain functions and mood. But when they are high, they can drive cholesterol into your artery walls and damage them. An optimal LDL level would be less than 100. 100–129 is above optimal, 130–159 is borderline, 160–189 is high, and anything greater than 190 is very high.

Bad cholesterol is elevated by the wrong diet, lack of exercise, and obesity. If LDL remains high, have your LDL particle size evaluated to see if you have good large fluffy particles or bad small dense particles.

HDL
HDL is known as good cholesterol. This is cholesterol that goes out of your arteries to be eliminated by your liver. A level less than 40 is low and a level greater than 60 is desirable.

Causes of low HDL include elevated triglycerides, obesity, lack of physical activity, type 2 diabetes, smoking, high carbohydrate intake (greater than 60%), and certain drugs (beta blockers, anabolic steroids, progestational agents).

Triglycerides
Your triglyceride level should be less than 100; the lower, the better. Triglycerides are different from other fats in that they are elevated by an excessive carbohydrate intake. You can decrease

this fat dramatically in a short time just by reducing your sugar and bad carb intake.

Ratios

Balance—in life and all areas of your body—is crucial. Therefore, it is important to look at the ratios of your numbers. Ratios are frequently more important than the individual numbers.

Total Cholesterol to HDL
The total cholesterol level itself is not the most important risk factor for heart disease. The ratio of total cholesterol to HDL is the number you should be concerned about. In general, the lower the ratio is, the lower your risk of heart attacks will be. Less than 2:1 is ideal, 4:1 is high, and 6:1 is very high risk.

Triglyceride to HDL
I believe this ratio is the most important predictor of heart disease. People with a high triglyceride level tend to have low HDL. Divide your triglycerides by your HDL level. If your result is 2 or less, that is considered ideal. 4 is high, and 6 is much too high. The lower this number is, the lower your risk of heart disease will be.

One study from a Harvard author said that high triglycerides alone increased the risk of heart attack by nearly three times, and people with the highest ratio of triglycerides to HDL had 16 times the risk of heart attack compared to those with the lowest ratio.

When my patients change to a healthy lifestyle, their LDL always gets lower, their HDL always gets higher, and their triglycerides always decrease. Each ratio that we have talked about can improve in a very short time.

Protein

To evaluate your blood protein, you should take a panel of tests that measure your total protein, albumin, globulin, and the albumin to globulin ratio.

Ideally, your total protein will be approximately 7.2–8.0 g/100 ml. Total protein may be elevated due to chronic infection, liver dysfunction, or dehydration.

It may be decreased due to insufficient intake and/or digestion of proteins, insufficient production of proteins from the liver, loss of protein through the GI tract from diarrhea, or loss through the urine in severe kidney disease.

What is more important than the total protein, though, are the individual levels of albumin and globulin.

Albumin

Albumin keeps blood from leaking out of your blood vessels. It also carries substances through the blood and is essential for tissue growth and healing. Albumin is produced in the liver using dietary protein. Your albumin is tested to see if your diet contains enough protein, to check that your kidneys and liver are working, and to determine why you have swelling or fluid retention. It is a very strong predictor of health.

The optimal range for albumin is 4.5–5.0 g/100 ml. Your albumin level may be elevated due to dehydration, heart failure, or poor protein utilization. Your level may be decreased by hypothyroidism, chronic debilitating diseases, protein deficiency, drinking too much water, kidney problems, diarrhea, or liver dysfunction.

Globulin

Globulin is made up of different proteins. Some globulins are made by the liver and others are made by the immune system. Globulins transport metals (such as iron) in the blood and help fight infection. Your globulin is tested to determine your chances of developing an infection, see if you have a blood disease, and check kidney and liver function.

The optimal range is 2.3–2.8 g/dL. Your globulin level may be elevated by chronic infections, liver disease, autoimmune disease, kidney dysfunction, and more. It may be decreased by kidney or liver disease.

Carbohydrates and Blood Sugar

There are four good tests to see how your body is handling sugar and carbohydrates.

Fasting Glucose

Ideally, your fasting glucose level should be 85 mg/dL or less. For every point above that, your risk of diabetes increases. If your glucose is 100, you will develop diabetes if you do not make changes. At 128, you are a diabetic.

Hemoglobin A1C

Hemoglobin A1C is a better test for blood sugar than fasting blood sugar because it gives you a three-month average of your blood sugar. Your values should be about 5. If you are at 6, that means you're diabetic. 7 means that your diabetes is out of control.

An A1C level of 5 means that your average blood sugar for the last three months was 97. 6=128, and 7=154.

Triglycerides

Triglycerides are a blood fat that increases when you consume too many bad carbohydrates. Your level should be less than 100 mg/dL but ideally closer to 50.

Fasting Insulin

This is my favorite of the four tests.

Your fasting insulin level should be lower than 5 mIU/L. Anything above that indicates that you're taking in too many bad carbohydrates. Remember, insulin is the key that unlocks the door to let glucose into your cells so that they get the energy they need. If your fasting insulin level is high, it indicates that your cells are becoming resistant to insulin and not allowing glucose in.

The overconsumption of high-GI foods drives up your blood sugar, insulin, and hemoglobin A1C, leading to metabolic syndrome and, eventually, diabetes. Eat lower-GI foods frequently and high-GI foods very sparingly.

4

The Energy System Mitochondria: Your Power Source

To go fast, you need a well-tuned, big engine.

Startling Facts:

- Lack of energy is one of the top symptoms that people mention when they visit a doctor.
- The risk for fatigue in women is about 1.5 times the risk for men, and the risk for people who do not exercise is twice that of active people.
- Lack of energy often indicates an underlying health problem.[1]

> *"Even if you're on the right track, you'll get run over if you just sit there."*
> —Will Rogers

Let's imagine that your other three Systems have been working correctly up to this point:

- Your Structural System is supported with real food.
- Your Digestive System broke the food down into small nutrients.
- Your Delivery System picked up the nutrients and delivered them to the cells.

Now that the cells have the nutrients they need, let's dive into the Energy System where those nutrients are turned into energy.

A Brief Introduction to The Energy System

Research shows that most diseases today start with the dysfunction of the Energy System.

The Energy System takes the nutrients delivered to the cells and turns them into energy that is used to power all the Systems of the body. If this System is not producing adequate energy, all the other Systems will sputter. Consider what happens when a power plant goes down—the whole region is plunged into darkness.

Many times, this "power outage" happens without us even knowing it. We ease into decreased energy production over many years, and we forget what having energy feels like. Look around. Everyone seems to be tired. Many of my patients come to me after they've seen many health professionals for issues related to a lack of energy.

Without a healthy supply of energy, we are unable to make proper decisions. As a result, every facet of our lives is affected—emotional, relational, spiritual, *and* physical.

If you constantly feel drained, there are probably deeper issues going on beneath the surface—on the cellular level. Until you address these underlying problems, you'll keep sabotaging your health efforts. Thankfully, you can reverse chronic weariness quickly with the 7 Systems Plan. In fact, you'll discover how to increase your energy up to 600%!

7 Signs That Your Energy System Is Working Against You:

1. Weight gain
2. Low energy, fatigue, or not feeling rested after a good night's sleep
3. Brain fog or forgetfulness
4. Getting winded easily
5. Headaches
6. Loss of smell or taste
7. Just plain feeling old

Meet Betty

One afternoon, an overweight woman in her mid-70s shuffled into my office. Although she had a pleasant smile, there was no sparkle in her eye. In the first few minutes, she explained why.

In her own words, she had no energy. Although she often slept, she never felt rested. Betty had many chronic conditions like elevated blood sugar, cholesterol, and blood pressure. On top of all this, her family had noticed her increased forgetfulness. She had a poor diet, did not take vitamins, failed to exercise, and did not know how to fix her problems.

Her medical doctor had a solution: prescription medicine. It had started with one prescription and eventually increased to eight per day. Her reason for visiting me was clear—she just wanted to "feel good again."

I saw that she had all the signs of a malfunctioning Energy System.

I started Betty on a program much like the one described in this chapter. After she had worked with me for six months, her family doctor took her off all the prescription medications because she no longer needed them. Her blood pressure was normal, and so were her cholesterol, blood sugar, and thyroid levels. Her energy had gone up tremendously, and she no longer needed to nap. She'd gained muscle and lost 43 pounds of fat.

Betty regained her youthful body in a very short time and started enjoying life. She'd been a widow for many years, but she began to date again. She told her family and friends, "I wish I had done this when I was 40."

In this chapter, I will show you the tools that Betty used to experience a complete energy transformation.

Why Your Energy System Is Working Against You

Mitochondria are the key to your energy, metabolism, weight, and health. Healthy mitochondria increase exercise performance, muscle mass, and your overall lifespan. If you have an abundance of optimally functioning mitochondria, you'll have a fast metabolism and burn calories effectively. On the other hand, mitochondrial dysfunction is linked to aging, diabetes, heart disease, fibromyalgia, chronic fatigue syndrome, schizophrenia, and depression.[2]

Your body's energy production process is called oxidative phosphorylation. This process produces adenosine triphosphate (ATP), which is used by the body for energy. We could get bogged down in the science of all this, so let me simplify it.

Your body takes in food (fuel), breaks it down in your Digestive System, and transports it to your cells. The nutrients enter the cells and are taken to the mitochondria.

Mitochondria are like microscopic power plants inside your cells. They generate 95% of your energy. In these power plants, fat and carbohydrates combine with oxygen to produce energy that powers your cells, your organs, and your entire body.

Mitochondria Facts

These tiny power plants produce 110 pounds of energy (ATP) per day. That's 10,000 times more energy production (pound for pound) than the sun. Each one of your cells may have several hundred or several thousand mitochondria. You could have as many as 10 million billion of them in your body, making up 10% of your body weight. It makes sense that the heart has the most mitochondria—5,000 per cell—because it is always working.

Mitochondria provide the energy that drives all cellular processes, including bringing nutrients into the cell, waste elimination, repair, and addressing problems. This last step includes making sure a cell self-destructs when it becomes abnormal or cancerous. Many experts believe that mitochondrial malfunction plays a major role in our cancer epidemic today.[3]

I make it a point to listen to my patients. I often hear them say, "No matter what I do, I cannot lose weight." When they say that, I look for a mitochondrial problem. If mitochondria are unprotected, poorly functioning, or low in number, the result is a slow metabolism and low energy. In this situation, you can't burn many calories, and you can't lose weight. You can solve this problem when you discover how to protect your mitochondria, supply them with what they need, and create more of them.

Let's continue our journey by utilizing a car analogy. How do you get the best performance out of your car?

Protect It

No one would purchase an expensive race car and fail to change the oil, oil filters, air filters, and tires. Taking these precautions protects the car from damage. Unfortunately, many people protect their cars better than they protect their bodies. The 7 Systems Plan will give you the tools you need to protect your mitochondria.

Give It Quality Fuel

If you put low-octane fuel in a race car, it will sputter and perform poorly regardless of how big the motor is. The same is true for your body. It is a high-performance biochemical machine that requires high-octane fuel to produce optimal energy and experience peak performance.

In the first three chapters, you discovered what you should eat and what you should avoid. Low-octane foods like white sugar, white flour, white bread, potatoes, fruit juice, junk food, and bad fats impair your body's performance.

Eating sugary food results in weight gain, inflammation, pain, and poor sleep. One junk food meal can decrease blood flow to all your vital organs and muscles by 25% for several hours.[4] Like a car, your body will sputter. When mitochondria fail to produce energy, all of your Systems suffer.

High-octane foods like vegetables, fruits, good fats, nuts, legumes, and quality proteins help your body perform at peak capacity. The effects of implementing the 7 Systems Plan are significant, and they're usually noticeable within 7–10 days.

Add A Bigger Motor

To increase a car's performance, you can add a supercharger or even put in a bigger motor. God created your body with amazing abilities. Not only can you supercharge your mitochondria and make them bigger, but you can also double the number in each cell.

If you know how, you can significantly increase the power produced by the mitochondria in your body. Every patient you've met so far—Mary, Jennifer, Ray, Betty—and those you will meet in the next few chapters discovered how to turn their bodies into a "ball of energy" by optimizing their mitochondrial function.

The 7 Systems Plan shows you three ways to double your mitochondria and optimize their function to give you unbelievable energy:

1. Protect your mitochondria.
2. Give your mitochondria what they need.
3. Direct your body to produce more mitochondria.

How to Get Your Energy System Working for You

Making your Energy System work for you and not against you involves a simple three-step process.

Step 1: Protect your mitochondria from free radical damage.

"Free radical" may conjure up visions of a hippie at Woodstock back in the '60s, but that is not what I mean.

What exactly is free radical damage? Oxygen in your body

can split into single atoms with unpaired electrons called free radicals. These single electrons want to pair up, so they bombard your cells, protein, and DNA, which causes damage.

Let me give you a couple of examples. If you leave metal out in the rain, water and oxygen will combine to rust the metal. If you cut an apple, it will turn brown. These are the effects of a process called oxidation, also known as free radical damage.

Free radicals can damage your mitochondria in the same way they damage the metal and the apple—they make you "rust" (age faster and lose energy).

Free radicals enter your body daily through water, air, and food, and they also form inside your body. They attack your cells every second and can compromise your cell membranes, causing them to become brittle and leak. They can also damage or kill your mitochondria. When this happens, your energy goes down and your cellular health and defenses suffer.

But if you take a sliced apple and dip it in lemon juice, it takes much longer to turn brown. This is the effect of antioxidants in the lemon that neutralize the free radicals. Antioxidants protect your mitochondria.

Antioxidants are your allies.
Antioxidants grab on to free radicals and neutralize them so they can be eliminated from your body without damaging you. These "allies" are found in certain vitamins (like C and E), some minerals (selenium), flavonoids from plants, and phytonutrients from fruits and vegetables.

CoQ10 is a great antioxidant that protects mitochondria from free radical damage and mops up potentially harmful byproducts created during energy production. It also facilitates the conversion of nutrients and oxygen into the energy that your cells need for life, repair, and regeneration.

Phytonutrients are your friends.
Phytonutrients from fruits and vegetables not only protect your mitochondria but also change how your cells function.

Remember, food is information that tells your cells what to do. This information can make your cells work better or worse. Phytonutrients from fruits and vegetables provide information that increases energy and decreases disease.

Eight out of ten Americans are deficient in phytonutrients such as lutein, indoles, chlorophyll, folate, beta-carotene, bioflavonoids, lycopene, resveratrol and many more.[5] These deficiencies cause 15,000 deaths per year and increase the risk of all chronic diseases including obesity, heart disease, cancer, hypertension, and stroke. How much does it help to add phytonutrients? You can lower your stroke risk by 26% simply by eating five servings of fruit and vegetables per day.[6]

Besides proper eating, you can also protect your mitochondria by controlling stress and getting adequate sleep. Failing to do so can make your mitochondria commit suicide—literally. In Chapter Five, you'll discover many helpful tools for proper stress management and sleep.

Phytonutrient Facts[7]

- Phytonutrients give fruits and vegetables their colors.
- 80% of all Americans have a "phytonutrient gap."
- 69% fall short in green phytonutrients, which helps vision and decreases cataracts and macular degeneration.
- 78% fall short in red, which reduces the risk of prostate, breast, and skin cancer as well as heart attacks.
- 86% fall short in white, which lowers cholesterol and helps the heart.
- 88% fall short in purple/blue, which decreases the risk of cancer, memory loss, diabetes, heart attacks, and Alzheimer's disease.
- 79% fall short in yellow/orange, which boosts immunity, decreases cancer and risk of heart attacks, and helps vision.

Step 2: Supply your mitochondria with quality nutrients.

By following the 7 Systems Plan, you'll give your mitochondria the building materials they need to function properly. Without key macronutrients, these power plants cannot work right, and your body cannot make more of them.

Be aware: Statins and antibiotics can damage mitochondria and should be used with caution. Also, too many calories and late-night eating overload the mitochondria and damage them. Restricting calories will make your mitochondria function better.

Eating close to bedtime damages your mitochondria. The calories that are not used while you sleep can back up in the mitochondria and harm them. Try not to eat for at least three hours before you go to bed. Taking this time off from eating will also help your mitochondria by "purging" them so they can function better. Try the FMD methods I shared in Chapter One.

Your mitochondria also need micronutrients, especially minerals, vitamins B and C, and amino acids, including taurine, L-carnitine, and malic acid. For my patients with significant mitochondrial dysfunction, I suggest a product called Cellular Energy which contains all of the above (see end of chapter for further information).

Step 3: Exercise to force your body to make more mitochondria.

Although nutrition is a vital part of ramping up mitochondrial function, exercise may be even more important. Exercise forces your body to produce more mitochondria so that it can keep up with the heightened energy requirements.

Dr. Jeffrey S. Bland, at the sixth annual Institute for Functional Medicine Symposium, stated that exercise doubles the number of power-producing mitochondria in the cells. It also increases power-producing enzymes by 300%. The result is a 600% energy increase. Imagine yourself with 600% more energy! How would your life be different?

According to the Centers for Disease Control and Prevention, 80% of Americans do not get enough exercise each week.[8] Proper exercise is not important only for mitochondria; researchers have found that exercise deficiency leads to obesity, type 2 diabetes, Alzheimer's disease, hypertension, and osteoporosis.[9] How much does not exercising affect your health? Studies show that failing to exercise may be as harmful to your health as smoking.[10]

The rest of the chapter will focus on exercise because you need to understand how to work *smarter*, not harder, in this area.

People think about exercise differently. Some love it. Some hate it. Many people think about exercise in the wrong way and believe common myths like the ones I've listed below. Debunking these myths will make your workouts more enjoyable. As a result, you'll have the energy to accomplish your goals.

Myth #1: Exercise depletes your energy.

When you exercise correctly, your Energy System (mitochondria) gets bigger and stronger. To test this, scientists examined cells under a microscope. By counting the number of mitochondria in different people's cells, they discovered the following facts:

- Inactive people had very few mitochondria.
- Those who walked regularly had more mitochondria.
- Those involved in aerobic exercise had even more mitochondria.
- Those with the most mitochondria were involved in regular aerobics, interval training, and weight lifting.[11]

Exercise actually produces more and more energy instead of the other way around. If you start small and make a habit of working out, your body will become an energy snowball, gathering more and more mitochondria to fuel more activity. You will feel much better, your weight will go down, and this will motivate you to continue to stay active.

Myth #2: Exercise wears down your body.

Actually, researchers have found the relationship between fitness level and mortality to be the exact opposite:

- Obesity + no exercise = one of the worst outcomes.
- Obesity + exercise (even without weight loss) = a much better outcome.
- No obesity + exercise = optimal health and outcome

It appears that exercise eliminates many of the negative effects of obesity.

Scientific studies show that regular exercise has the following benefits:

- Increases energy, longevity, strength, balance, and endurance
- Enhances immune and brain function and protects against dementia
- Decreases the risk of infections
- Lowers the risk of all forms of cardiovascular disease (high blood pressure, heart attacks, strokes, elevated cholesterol, etc.)
- Protects against cancers
- Reduces stress and inflammation
- Relieves anxiety, elevates mood, prevents and treats depression
- Improves quality of sleep
- Increases sexual function and frequency by 33%
- Protects against type 2 diabetes and osteoporosis

Myth #3: Exercise is of limited value if you have heart disease.

In Germany, researchers studied patients with heart disease. Half of the group got a stent (coronary angioplasty), and the other half got an exercise program.[12]

After one year, 88% of the exercise group was event-free (no heart attack) compared to only 70% of the stent group. Exercise benefited all the arteries of the body while the stent benefited only the one artery.

Another group studied several hundred thousand people between 1996 and 2008. They found that a mere 15 minutes of exercise per day could increase your lifespan by 3 years. Those who got themselves moving for at least 15 minutes per day or 90 minutes per week also had a 14% reduced risk for all causes of mortality.[13]

Myth #4: Walking will hardly change anything.

Only one hour of walking per week decreases your chances of dying by 20%. Two and a half hours per week decreases your chances of dying by 30%.

A study was done in Japan to find out how walking to work affected blood pressure.[14] Here is what they found:

- Walking for 10 minutes showed no improvement.
- Walking for 11–20 minutes decreased high blood pressure risk by 12%.
- Walking over 20 minutes decreased high blood pressure risk by 29%.

For every additional 10 minutes of walking to work, there was a 12% decrease in the chances of getting high blood pressure.

Exercise is the number one treatment for fatigue. It gives you the biggest return on investment, and it's been shown to help more health problems than almost anything else. Look at the benefits people get just by walking:

- 47% decrease in arthritis pain and disability
- 50% decreased progression of dementia and Alzheimer's
- 58% decrease in prediabetes progressing to diabetes
- 41% decreased risk of hip fracture in older women
- 48% decrease in anxiety
- 50% decrease in heart disease
- 47% decreased depression

Many studies show that cancer patients who exercise regularly decrease the reoccurrence rate significantly compared to non-exercisers. Remember that exercise ramps up mitochondria. The evidence strongly indicates that exercise should be included in the standard of care for cancer.[15]

Myth #5: You need to eat before exercise.

Many people think that they cannot work out on an empty stomach. Your body does need fuel to work out—fuel, but not food. Remember from Chapter One that when your body does not have food or stored carbohydrates, it is forced to switch over to burning stored fat.

Three days a week, I play tennis from 11:30 to 1:00. My first meal of the day comes after that. Since I started practicing time-restricted eating, my energy has gone up significantly. I have more endurance. I don't get winded as easily. And I play better tennis.

You will burn more body fat when you exercise if you do not eat beforehand. However, it is important to eat within 30 minutes of completing a strenuous workout. Taking a quality protein will help you build more muscle.

Some amino acids are essential to build muscle; leucine, for example. Leucine is found in meat, dairy, eggs, and pea and rice protein isolate. Some experts think you need 1–3 grams of leucine per day to build and maintain muscle. See my recommendation for quality protein at the end of this chapter.

Myth #6: Exercise is more important than diet for weight loss.

Your diet is by far the biggest factor in weight loss. You simply cannot out-exercise your mouth. Linking the calories in a product to the amount of exercise required to burn them off can give you a healthy perspective:

- 20-ounce soft drink = walk 4.5 miles
- Large combo meal = jog 4 miles a day for a week

However, exercise influences your Systems so much that it is essential. It has been called the ultimate lever for optimal weight and health.

We now know that exercise boosts a fat-burning hormone called irisin (a.k.a. FNDC5). This hormone not only helps your body burn fat but also keeps fat cells from forming in the first place. It can suppress fat cell formation by 20–60%.[16]

Exercise Tips

As you exercise, your muscle mass increases and body fat decreases. This is the reverse of what normally happens as you age. Fitness (muscle mass) is the single biggest indicator of health in old age. If you have lost it, you must regain it. Here is what you should do to make exercise more enjoyable and effective.

- **Do it long enough:** In general, more is better, but the benefits of exercise seem to decrease after about 30 minutes per day. The higher the intensity, the less time you need. The lower intensity, the more time you need.
- **Do something you enjoy:** What do you enjoy doing? What could you start doing that you might enjoy? Walk with a friend, join an exercise group, put your treadmill in front of the TV, or listen to music while you exercise (this burns up to 15% more calories). If you can do something you enjoy, it will be much easier to continue long-term, but even if you don't enjoy exercise, you need to do it. Even the great exercise guru Jack LaLanne said that he did not like to work out, but he liked what it did to him. You will soon love what it does to you.
- **Do focus on how much better you feel:** Dopamine is a reward neurotransmitter released in the brain when you experience something enjoyable. Many people have an increase in dopamine secretion during exercise. You may have heard of the "runners high." If you haven't experienced this, there is hope. You can "rewire" your brain so

that exercise becomes pleasurable and rewarding. Focusing on how much better you feel is a great motivator to continue.

- **Do it correctly:** Take baby steps. The perfect starter exercise routine should include 5 minutes of stretching, 10 minutes of strength training or weight lifting, and 30 minutes of an aerobic exercise at least 3 times per week. You can make tremendous improvements in your health by doing this simple routine.

Stretching

As we get older, we lose our range of motion and our joints become stiff. If you want to stay healthy, recover your flexibility by stretching. Focus on five major areas when you stretch:

1. Neck
2. Shoulders
3. Back
4. Hips
5. Legs

This routine should only take you about five minutes. Go to 7SystemsPlan.com to see how to perform these stretches safely.

To stretch, all you need to do is move the joint to the end of its range of motion and hold it for three seconds. Do not bounce, and do not go too far. If you have lost flexibility, it will take time to get it back.

Weight Lifting

Weight lifting is the only way to increase muscle mass significantly. To be honest, it is something I don't enjoy as much as tennis. However, since I started weight lifting with my son, it's become something I look forward to. It's always more fun to work out with other people, and group weight lifting tends to make us work harder than we would alone. After all, people are watching.

A good weight lifting routine involves several muscle groups with 10 repetitions and 3 sets of each exercise. Work one muscle group and then go to the next and the next without stopping. In Appendix A, Part Seven, I show you how to work more than one muscle group at the same time to shorten your workout.

Again, I provide sample routines at 7SystemsPlan.com that work most muscles in the body in an easy 10-minute workout. Very few people want to lift weights for an hour, but most can handle 10 minutes. If done correctly, 10 minutes can benefit your body tremendously.

Aerobic

In general, you need to do something that raises your pulse rate for 30 minutes at least 3 times per week. If you are trying to lose weight, you should do it 5 times per week. For maximum benefit, you need to get your heart rate up into the target zone (see chart in Appendix A, Part Seven). It does not matter what you do as long as it gets your pulse into your target zone.

One way you'll know that your heart is in the target zone is if you are slightly breathless. You should not be able to carry on a normal conversation without having to take a breath every few words. See how easy it is to say "Mary had a little lamb whose fleece was white as snow" while exercising. If you can do it without taking a breath, you are not in the zone. It should be more like this: "Mary had a (breath) little lamb (breath) whose fleece was white (breath) as snow."

Get good at checking your pulse. Reach around your wrist and put your fingers on your forearm below your thumb. You should feel a pulse. If you prefer another method, reach across your neck and slide to the center to find your carotid artery.

Count your pulse for six seconds and then add a zero to get your heart beats per minute. Work toward being able to keep your pulse in your target zone the entire 30 minutes to get the most from the exercise. (Appendix A, Part Seven). Exercising below your target zone has limited benefit.

Most people know that they burn more calories when they exercise. However, most people don't know that if you exercise in your aerobic zone for 30 minutes, you increase your metabolism and the calories you burn for many hours after the exercise stops. This can result in a significant number of calories burned and greater weight loss.

Interval Training

Studies have shown that some types of exercise create more mitochondria than others. Interval training seems to outdo all others.[17]

Interval training is moderate aerobic exercise with short bursts of intense exercise at specific times. This training triggers mitochondrial biogenesis, which is important for both energy and longevity. One review in *Applied Physiology, Nutrition, and Metabolism* showed that interval training alters mitochondrial enzyme content and activity, which helps increase energy production. This also decreases your risk of chronic disease and slows down the aging process.[18]

Consider the following aerobic riddle:

Question: Which is more beneficial—50 minutes of biking or 10 minutes of biking that includes three 20-second bursts of intense biking?

Answer: They are equally beneficial.

Short, intense bursts of exercise do amazing things to your body! Although you can do many variations of intervals, I suggest a 20-minute aerobic session with a 30-second burst of exercise every 2 minutes. Some activities like tennis and basketball are naturally interval training.

Here are the three keys to getting maximum results from exercise: intensity, intensity, intensity. Work up to the point where you can incorporate intense bursts into your workout.

A recent study in the *Journal of Obesity* found that 12 weeks of interval training significantly reduced abdominal, trunk, and visceral fat. It also significantly increased aerobic power (maximal oxygen uptake, or VO_2max).[19]

In another study, young overweight males were either assigned to an interval training exercise group or a control exercise group.[20] The results were impressive. The interval training was conducted for 20 minutes 3 times a week for 3 months. Compared to the control group, the interval group had an additional 4.4 pounds of weight loss and 17% reduction in visceral or abdominal fat.

Benefits of Interval Training:

- 20 minutes of interval training benefits you more than 40 minutes of aerobic exercise.
- Interval training burns 33% more fat than aerobic exercise.
- Each interval training session may increase your growth hormone levels by 771%! Human growth hormone (HGH) is the miracle youth hormone that makes you younger. As we get older, our HGH declines. Interval training is one of the few types of exercise that can boost HGH.[21]

Beginner Intervals:
Walk for 90 seconds, then power walk (walk fast and swing your arms) for 30 seconds. Slow down and recover for 90 seconds, then do another 30-second burst.

At first, you may only be able to do 2 or 3 bursts during the 20-minute session. As you become fit, add more bursts until you get up to 8 during the 20-minute workout.

Intermediate Intervals:
Power walk for 90 seconds, jog for 30 seconds, and repeat.

Advanced Intervals:
Jog for 90 seconds, run as fast as you can for 30 seconds, and repeat.

You can do interval training with biking, a treadmill, an elliptical machine, swimming—just about anything. The good news is that you only need to do it for 20 minutes.

Do interval training every other day so that your body has time to recover. You can download interval timers on your phone to keep track of the time for you. Visit 7SystemsPlan.com for a variety of free apps.

Remember this word of caution: Interval training is for people who have been doing aerobic exercise for some time and are proficient at it. If you have heart problems or other health issues, you should not try interval training without your doctor's consent.

In my office, I teach a class that combines nonstop weight lifting and interval training. We do 90 seconds of weight lifting followed by a 30-second burst of more intense exercise like jumping jacks, burpees, or running in place. This fits both weight lifting and interval training into a 20-minute workout. See Appendix A, Part Seven, for more information.

Pedometers

Studies[22] show that putting on a pedometer will

- Increase your steps per day by 2,491
- Decrease your systolic blood pressure by 3.8 mmHg
- Reduce your weight by .4%

Make sure you put it on your body correctly, and do not buy the cheapest model. You should spend at least $15–20.

I prefer watches that monitor your heart rate and pulse. My article on 7SystemsPlan.com lists some suggested models.

Sex

People who exercise have significantly more sex and sex is a form of exercise![23] During sex, your body has an increased heart rate, increased blood pressure, and slightly increased perspiration. The aerobic benefit is equivalent to walking two miles per hour or doing light housework. However, since most sexual encounters do not last long, you are not going to get much exercise out of it.

But orgasm is a different story.

During orgasm, your heart rate can rise above 130 beats per minute, your blood pressure can elevate to 170 systolic, and your perspiration can be profuse. This is the equivalent of walking three to four miles per hour or, for some, an all-out run. The effect is similar to interval training.

Sex has other health benefits. Queens University in Belfast tracked 1,000 middle-aged men for over 10 years. Those who had orgasms twice per week or more had half as many heart attacks.[24] Sex, like intense exercise, can increase human growth hormone levels.[25]

Quick Recap:

- Mitochondrial health is the key to your health.
- Mitochondria produce 95% of your energy. Protect them and give them the right fuel.
- Certain types of exercise will increase the number of mitochondria in your body and give you 600% more energy.
- You will lose more weight if you exercise on an empty stomach.
- Muscles, tendons, and joints benefit from stretching.
- Weight lifting is the only significant way to increase muscle mass.
- Aerobic exercise has great benefits.
- Interval training produces maximum health benefits.

- You can combine weight lifting and interval training to compress a workout into 20 minutes for maximum efficiency.

Proven Steps to Fix Your Energy System:

(Check these off as you complete them. Join our free 7 Systems Plan Community for additional support and encouragement: 7SystemsPlan.com.)

☐ Support and protect your mitochondria with vital macronutrients and micronutrients.

☐ Stretch, lift weights, and start walking daily (work your way up to 30 minutes).

☐ Try integrating interval training into your exercise regimen (if you're cleared by your doctor).

Supplements to Support Your Energy System

The functional food that Betty used to support her Energy System, rebuild her muscle, and lose weight was Dynamic Daily Meal. It supplies nutritional support for age-related muscle loss. Since Betty had significant mitochondrial impairment, she also used a product called Cellular Energy for mitochondria and cell function support. See Appendix A, Part Five, or 7SystemsPlan.com for more information.

Energy System Lab Tests

Simple At-Home Test: Measure Your Fitness Level.

See how many pushups, sit-ups, and squats you can do in one minute. See Appendix A, Part Seven, or go to 7SystemsPlan. com. I provide several examples of assessments that measure your upper and lower body strength, abdominal strength, explosive power, aerobic endurance, and flexibility. Track your improvement once a month.

If you have a functional medicine doctor, ask for the following tests:

- Bioimpedance Analysis—shows your pounds of muscle and fat and your cellular health
- KORR Metabolic Testing—an exact measurement of your metabolism

5

The Communication System Hormones, Nerves, and Neurotransmitters

Good health results from good communication.

Startling Facts

- 1 in 4 men over age 30 has low testosterone.[1]
- An estimated 20 million Americans have some form of thyroid disease, and up to 60% of them are unaware of their condition.[2]
- 90% of adults over age 50 have a problem with their hormones, nerves, or neurotransmitters.

> *"In the 21st century, our taste buds, our brain chemistry, our biochemistry, our hormones and our kitchens have been hijacked by the food industry."*
> —Mark Hyman

Let's imagine that your other four Systems have been working correctly up to this point:

- Your Structural System is supported with real food.
- Your Digestive System broke the food down into small nutrients.
- Your Delivery System picked up the nutrients and delivered them to the cells.
- Your Energy System (mitochondria) turned the nutrients into energy.

What you need next is a way for all the Systems to communicate for optimal functionality.

A Brief Introduction to The Communication System

For your first four Systems to work together at the same time, they must talk to each other. This is where your Communication System comes into play. It has three main players:

1. Hormones
2. Nerves
3. Neurotransmitters

In this chapter, we'll discover how your Systems communicate. When the Communication System is working correctly, you'll lose weight, heal chronic illness, and reverse aging.

Hormones

The word hormone comes from the Greek word *hormon*, which means to excite or set in motion. Hormones are essential for the proper function of each of the body's Systems. Your body has 80+ different hormones, and they all perform different tasks. They control everything from your body temperature to your appetite.

Many factors can disrupt your hormones, including weight,

diet, stress, aging, drugs, and chemicals in the environment. You can optimize or impair them by what you do to your body.

Nerves

Nerves transfer electrical impulses from the brain to the Systems. These impulses are instructions telling the Systems what to do. Separate nerves carry signals back to the brain, giving it feedback. If you've ever touched a hot plate, you've pulled your hand back because of your nerves. Sensory nerves feel the heat and signal the brain, and the brain sends signals back through the motor nerves to let go of the plate—all in less than one second. Optimal electrical flow through your nerves is a critical part of your Communication System.

Neurotransmitters (NTs)

The 46 miles of nerves in your body are not in one long, continuous string. You have billions of separate nerves with junctions or gaps between them. Your brain and gut produce chemical messengers called neurotransmitters (NTs) to transfer signals between these nerves. Your brain uses NTs to tell the Systems what to do. They can make your heart beat faster, your lungs breathe quicker, and your stomach speed up or slow down digestion. NTs also have a significant effect on your mood.

7 Signs That Your Communication System Is Working Against You:

1. Weight gain
2. Night sweats or feeling cold
3. Low morning energy or loss of sex drive
4. More stress than you can handle
5. Depression or sleep problems
6. High blood sugar or high blood pressure
7. Back or neck pain or numbness and tingling

Meet Donna

Donna, a 55-year-old, walked into my office dressed warmer than the weather demanded. She complained about back pain. By her own admission, she didn't feel her "normal" self. Her energy was low, her sleep conflicted, and her sex life nonexistent. She suffered from weight gain, mild depression, diabetes, and she was on medication. To top it off, she felt cold most of the time. (That explained the sweater.)

During my examination, I noticed that she had lost the outer third of her eyebrow, her hair was thinning, and the skin on the back of her hands was thin. Lab test showed high thyroid-stimulating hormone (sign of an underactive thyroid), high HbA1C (sign of diabetes), high fasting insulin level (sign of insulin resistance), and low vitamin D. Spinal evaluation and X-rays revealed significant subluxations in both her cervical and lumbar spine. It was clear that Donna's Communication System was working against her.

She began using the 7 Systems Plan, specifically the steps found in this chapter. After 90 days, Donna had experienced a radical transformation. She had acquired newfound energy, was much happier, lost 35 pounds, gained visible muscle, and reached her ideal weight. Spinal adjustments restored vertebral alignment and optimized nerve function. For the first time in a long time, her back felt better. The condition of her hair and skin improved significantly, and most of her symptoms disappeared.

Her HbA1C decreased from 7.2 to 5.5, indicating that her diabetes was gone. Her thyroid level returned to normal. Her vitamin D rose from 18 to 52, and her insulin dropped from 23 to 5.

However, she continued to have decreased libido and sleep problems. She would frequently lay awake for two hours before drifting off to sleep. Further testing revealed that her progesterone, testosterone, and estrogen were low because of her age and a hysterectomy.

Since Donna had already been working on the 7 Systems Plan, exercise, and stress control, she was a perfect candidate for bioidentical hormone replacement therapy (BHRT). Her response to treatment was impressive. Within a few days, she was going to sleep immediately, her energy picked up even more, and her libido increased.

You can experience the same benefits if you follow the steps in this chapter.

Hormones

Hormones are an important part of your health. They are like army generals traveling through your bloodstream, telling cells and Systems what to do. Some of these hormones are five-star generals—they control other hormones. Some have long careers and work throughout your lifetime (thyroid hormone). Others retire early and slow down when you are in your early twenties (growth hormone). When a general arrives at its target site (the receptor site where it attaches to the cell), it changes the way that cell or System performs. It can make it work harder or force it to rest.

These generals are very powerful, but they can be rendered ineffective by poor lifestyle choices and outside influences that lower their numbers and block receptor sites. I am going to teach you how to optimize your hormone function and bring youth hormones out of retirement. When your hormones work well, it becomes easier to lose weight and feel young again.

You can have too little or too much of a hormone. A hormone deficiency impairs the function of all your other Systems. You'll experience grave consequences like weight gain, low energy, and disease. A hormone excess bombards your cells so that your receptor sites "tune out" and stop responding. An example of this is type 2 diabetes (insulin resistance).

We can also have imposters, like toxins, take the place of our hormones. Endocrine-disrupting chemicals like BPA and phthalates (found in plastics) are dangerous even in tiny amounts because they bind to your cells' receptor sites and block your hormones.

Your body has feedback pathways to regulate hormone production. When all of your hormones, receptor sites, and feedback pathways are working, life is good. When even one of these does not function properly, you can have serious problems.

Though there are over 80 hormones and hundreds of neurotransmitters working in your body, you only need to focus on a few important ones to get your Systems back in order.

First, we will explore what you need to keep your body functioning. Next, we'll explore what will take your life to a whole new level. After learning the information in this chapter, you will understand the hormones that contribute to weight gain, mood, sleep, focus, craving, memory, anxiety, and contentment.

Hormones that Keep You Alive

Two hormones form the foundation of your hormone Communication System.

Insulin: Why It's Working Against You

Insulin is your energy and fat storage hormone. It is produced in the pancreas, and it is classified as an anabolic hormone or building hormone. Its main purpose is to drive fuel either into cells for energy or fat for storage. You cannot fuel your cells or store fat without it. People with type 1 diabetes have no insulin; they can eat enormous amounts of food and still not gain weight. They must take insulin, or they will die.

A much more widespread problem is excess insulin, which leads to type 2 diabetes or insulin resistance syndrome. High insulin is associated with all five of the top killers in America:

1. Heart disease
2. Hypertension
3. Stroke
4. Cancer
5. Type 2 diabetes

Keeping your insulin at the ideal level significantly decreases your risk for all of these diseases. The longest living people have the lowest insulin (less than 5 mcIU/mL is ideal) and the most cellular sensitivity to insulin.

The #1 factor leading to increased insulin is consuming too many bad carbohydrates. You can turn this around fairly quickly when you pay attention to the type of carbohydrates you're eating. As we already discussed in Chapter Three, focus on eating low-GI carbohydrates and limiting the high-GI ones.

How Insulin Works

Sugar from digested carbohydrates (in the form of glucose) is the main fuel source for cells, but it cannot get into cells without insulin's assistance. Think of insulin as a key that opens the door to a cell—the sugar receptors. When you eat, your blood sugar goes up, and the pancreas responds by sending insulin to let sugar into your cells. When this happens, your blood sugar goes down to normal, your cells get energy, and your body is happy.

That is what happens when the Systems are all working correctly. However, when you eat too many bad carbohydrates, or even excess protein, your blood sugar increases more than it should. Since high blood sugar is toxic and damages your blood vessels, your pancreas responds to this crisis by making more insulin.

But more insulin does not always allow more sugar to get into a cell. If insulin is too high for too long, the receptors on the cell "tune out" the insulin and stop hearing it. If you have a friend who is constantly calling and texting you, what do you do? Eventually, you tune them out and stop listening. The same is true when insulin remains high for too long.

High levels of saturated fat inside the cell also "gum up" the lock on the cell. Fat from your diet or your body can build up in the cell and create toxic products that impair insulin's function.[3] If you keep sticking gum in the lock on your car door, eventually, the key will no longer work.

The death spiral caused by a poor diet and high insulin:

1. Insulin is too high, and glucose receptors on the cells respond by tuning out—they stop "listening."

2. Sugar that cannot get into the cells is converted into fat. The fat from your diet and body "gums up" the locks, and you gain weight.

3. Because blood sugar remains high, the pancreas releases more and more insulin in an attempt to drive more glucose into the cells.

4. Your muscle and fat cells are filled with even more fat, and they resist insulin more. You now have insulin resistance syndrome.

5. Sustained high insulin and blood sugar levels cause fat to accumulate in the liver, and before long, the liver becomes toxic and you develop fatty liver disease. Insulin function is impaired even more because of your liver, and now you have type 2 diabetes.

6. Eventually, the pancreas also becomes fatty and exhausted, and it quits working. Now you have type 1 diabetes.

Sadly, the medical community's usual answer to high blood sugar is a drug that drives even more glucose into the cells: insulin, sulphonylureas, or metformin. These drugs lower blood sugar but do not address the underlying pathophysiology of type 2 diabetes. The answer is not to drive more and more sugar into sick cells, but to change your diet to make your insulin work for you again.

Remember, when sugar cannot get into a cell, it is converted to fat for storage. As a result, your weight goes up. Elevated insulin is a significant factor in weight gain and makes it harder to lose weight. It's "fat fertilizer." High insulin causes fat cells to grow and blocks the release of fat. You can combat this effect by maintaining healthy levels of insulin in your bloodstream at all times.

How to Get Insulin Working for You

Lower your insulin by following these seven steps:

1. Eliminate high-GI foods and follow the eating guide in Chapters One and Three. You will not lower your insulin without decreasing your consumption of bad carbohydrates. This adjustment will solve most of your issues.
2. Do not overconsume protein and saturated fat. Instead, follow The 7 System Plan.
3. Reduce calories.
4. Reduce fructose; it increases insulin resistance 25% more than sucrose (table sugar).
5. Limit caffeinated beverages to two cups per day; caffeine stimulates insulin release.
6. Eliminate alcohol in the weight-loss phase; it is just another carbohydrate. Once you reach your ideal weight, women should have no more than one alcoholic beverage per day, and men should have no more than two.
7. Follow the suggestions in this chapter to eliminate stress.

Cortisol: Why It's Working Against You

Cortisol is your stress hormone. Almost all illness is caused by stress, aggravated by stress, or brings more stress. 25% of Americans rate their stress level between 8 and 10 on a 10-point scale.

According to the American Psychological Association, stress is linked to six of the leading causes of death:

1. Heart disease
2. Cancer
3. Lung ailments
4. Accidents
5. Cirrhosis
6. Suicide

It is the number one reason that people eat poorly, quit healthy lifestyle programs, and practice substance abuse.[4] You must deal with stress to lose weight and stay healthy.

Stress increases the production of cortisol by the adrenal glands that sit on top of the kidneys. It is the only hormone that increases with age. Cortisol is not bad in and of itself. It helps your body handle stress by ramping up your Systems' ability to fight or flee stressful events. It produces a similar effect to stepping on the gas pedal in your car.

Acute, short-term stress is a part of life and is necessary for survival. The problem comes when it's not short-term, but chronic. The overproduction of cortisol wreaks havoc on our Systems, destroys muscle, and encourages fat storage. Stress can also lead to bingeing on sugar-rich foods, which contributes to even more fat accumulation.

Referencing the car analogy again, think of the problems that can occur if you hold the gas pedal to the floor while it's in park. This is what happens when you are under chronic stress.

Dr. Robert M. Sapolsky gives an example of how the physiological stress response works:

> *"When [you're a zebra running] for your life, basics are all that matter. Lungs work overtime to pump mammoth quantities of oxygen into the bloodstream. The heart races to pump that oxygen throughout the body, so muscles respond instantly. You need your blood pressure up to deliver that energy. You need to turn off anything that's not essential . . . growth, reproduction . . . tissue repair, all of that sort of thing. Do it later if there is a later."*[5]

We now know that thoughts and everyday life events (psychological stress) can trigger the same stress response and its accompanying release of cortisol. Dr. Sapolsky continues:

> *"When the zebra escapes, its stress response shuts down, but human beings can't seem to find their off switch. We turn on the exact same stress response for purely psychological states. Thinking about the ozone layer, the taxes coming up, mortality, thirty-year mortgages—we turn on the same stress response, and the key difference there is we're not doing it for a real physiological reason, and we're*

doing it nonstop. After a while, the stress response is more damaging than the stressor itself because the stress is some psychological nonsense you're falling for. No zebra on earth running for its life would understand why fear of speaking in public would cause you to secrete the same hormones that it's doing at that point to save its life." [5]

Chronic stress—whether real or imagined—activates metabolic pathways that cause weight gain, high blood sugar, increased belly fat, high blood pressure, high cholesterol, muscle loss, insulin resistance, carbohydrate craving, decreased libido, gastrointestinal problems, anxiety, depression, and a slowing of your metabolism.

- Cortisol elevations increase your appetite and motivation to eat. If stress caused an increase in your appetite for vegetables, you would not have a problem. But stress seems to increase your appetite for foods that are high in sugar and fat. Eating these foods can make you feel better temporarily. They're called "comfort foods" for a reason.
- Chronic stress depletes your sex hormones. When you are under stress, your body shifts from making other hormones (testosterone, estrogen, progesterone) to making more cortisol.
- Chronic elevation of cortisol can result in cortisol resistance. If this continues and cortisol is elevated for too long, your adrenal glands wear down. This can lead to adrenal insufficiency, which brings a decline in function and increases aging.

If you want to lose weight and be healthy, you must control stress.[6]

Chronic and long-term stress not only makes you gain weight, but it also kills you. Studies show that chronic stress can shorten your life by 10 years!

How to Get Cortisol Working for You

Make your cortisol work for you by reducing stress. You can decrease stress in many ways, some of which we'll discuss below. Stress can be classified into four main categories:

1. Psychological Stressors
2. Environmental Stressors
3. Metabolic Stressors
4. Physiological Stressors

Let's unpack these one at a time.

Psychological Stressors:
You might have this kind of stress if you are experiencing family or work problems, unemployment, or financial difficulties, are obsessing over the past or future, too busy, or grieving the death of someone close to you.

We can overcome these stressors by fixing our thinking. Many people get into habits of thinking, beliefs, and ideas that keep them stressed. Practice mindfulness: controlling what your mind is thinking about.

Step 1: Mindfulness Meditation
Begin this process by sitting comfortably, focusing on your breathing, and bringing your mind's attention to the present moment without drifting into concerns about the past or the future. This form of meditation has enjoyed increasing popularity in recent years. Research suggests that it may be helpful for people with anxiety, depression, and pain.

You can meditate in many ways. I suggest you find a quiet, comfortable place and either sit or lie down. Quiet your mind and breathe deeply. I take a different approach to meditation than many Eastern religions. I do not suggest that you empty your mind and repeat a meaningless phrase over and over again.

I suggest that you use the time for prayer and thinking about things that are good and pure and lovely. Reciting a Bible verse works well. For example, try Psalm 23: "The Lord is my

Shepherd. . . ." You can substitute this with an inspirational quote if you do not read Scripture.

Do not allow your mind to wander, and if it does, come back to your meditation.

Step 2: Time Management
Gaining more control over your time is an important step in controlling stress. Make sure you set priorities, organize your day, and delegate what you can. Do not overschedule.

Let perfectionism go. Perfectionists have more trouble sticking to a weight-loss plan. Focus on progress, not perfection.

Step 3: Social Support and Community
Support from friends and family creates a buffering effect on your stress. We all need someone to talk to. Being around others can limit harmful or false thoughts. Isolation often exacerbates stress, while real relationships reduce psychological stress.

Environmental Stressors:
These stressors show up in the form of chemical or toxic exposure, infections, and annoying noise.

In Chapter Seven, you'll learn that toxins are a serious problem for most people. They can quickly overwhelm your Systems. Environmental stressors such as mercury from fish, BPA from plastic, chlorine from water, herbicides from food, and sugar are a few you need to eliminate. We will dive deep into environmental toxins in the next chapter. For now, I want you to identify your own stress-causing culprits.

Another environmental stress is poor oral hygiene. Dental problems are a common source of bacteria entering the body. These bacteria can trigger a chronic inflammatory stress response. If you have gum disease or receding gums, you must work with your dentist to correct these problems.

Try to limit your toxin exposure, eliminate infections, and silence annoying noises. Also, consider detoxifying your body (see Chapter Seven).

Metabolic Stressors:
These stressors include nutritional deficiencies, inflammation, obesity, insulin resistance, and free radical damage.

Your body may have metabolic stress long before you notice it. If this stress is not resolved, it will negatively affect your mood and your response to outward stress.

Step 1
Lose weight. Staying on the 7 Systems Plan is the best solution to your weight problems.

Step 2
Use micronutrients and herbs to decrease stress. I suggest the following:

- B-complex vitamins—these help your body handle stress.
- Folate—depression and anxiety can be related to poor folate metabolism. Note: Many people cannot convert folate to the active form, so use only the active form, methyltetrahydrofolate.
- Omega-3 EPA and DHA—75% of Americans have silent inflammation, a primary cause of stress in your body. Omega-3 can help silence inflammation.[7]
- Vitamin D3—this helps lower stress, depression, and cortisol.
- Herbal supplements—licorice root, holy basil, ashwagandha, passion flower, kava kava, St. John's wort, and lavender can modify your stress response.

Physiological Stressors:
You might have this kind of stress if you suffer from structural or spinal problems, trauma, pain, or poor sleep. Restoring correct spinal alignment and posture, eliminating pain, exercising, and improving sleep habits decreases physiological stress.

Step 1: Moderate-Intensity Exercise
Exercise is a vital part of any stress management program. Moderate-intensity exercise helps decrease cortisol. It is shown

to be more effective than drugs for treating mild to moderate depression. Choose an activity that leaves you refreshed and energized. After a two-week trial, you'll experience remarkable results.

Step 2: Vibration

Vibration is an incredibly effective way to lower stress. You can purchase vibrating exercise equipment, or you can experiment with an option that doesn't cost you any money.

Try standing up, rising on your toes, and then dropping down on your heels. This will send a vibration through your body. Repeat this as quickly as you can while you are relaxing your back, arms, neck, and shoulders. Let your hands flop and send this vibration throughout your body. Doing this for two minutes should lower your stress level.

You can get the same type of vibration benefit from regular exercise. When I play tennis, I vibrate my body by running, stopping, starting, and jumping.

Step 3: Power Postures

Power postures lower the stress response. Sitting or standing in a closed position (legs crossed, arms folded, bent forward) can increase your stress and stress hormones. The solution is to sit and stand in the power postures.

Sitting: Sit with your shoulders back, arms open, and legs apart.

Standing: The most powerful posture is the Wonder Woman position. Stand with your legs a little bit apart, shoulders back, and hands on your hips. Do not underestimate the power of this technique. According to Amy Cuddy of Harvard University, two minutes in this position can increase your testosterone and decrease cortisol by up to 20%!

Step 4: Sleep and Rest

Sleep and adequate rest are imperative. Your body needs to get enough sleep to heal, repair, and recuperate. If you are not getting seven to eight hours of sleep, you are damaging your body.

Sleep deprivation leads to accelerated aging and weight gain. The biological mechanisms linking sleep deprivation and weight gain are numerous. They include metabolic changes, altered insulin sensitivity, and altered stress mechanisms that negatively affect gene expression.

We'll address sleep in detail in the next chapter. Check out my tips for a good night's sleep at 7SystemsPlan.com.

Step 5: Deep Breathing
I have a few favorite relaxation techniques that I recommend, but the most helpful is diaphragmatic breathing. This can be practiced anywhere—at any time. You can do it while you are waiting in traffic, in a line, or for an appointment. And it does not cost a thing.

Andrew Wells teaches this technique in the following manner: Inhale through your nose to a count of four. Hold your breath for seven seconds and exhale through your mouth to a count of eight. When you inhale, breathe deeply into your abdomen and feel it expand as you count to four. Pause for a count of seven. Exhale, through your mouth slowly, to a count of eight, allowing the tension to release. Repeat this until you feel relaxed or for at least two minutes.

This is a powerful technique that should be used regularly. Studies have shown that it can decrease symptoms of depression significantly, at the same time boosting the level of gamma-aminobutyric acid (GABA), a calming neurotransmitter.[8]

Breathing exercises have also been shown to reduce salivary cytokines associated with inflammation and stress.[9]

Hormones that Give You Life

Leptin, thyroid, testosterone, estrogen, and progesterone are the five main hormones that help you thrive. You can live without these hormones, but life loses its appeal. When these minor hormones are in balance, they also protect against degenerative diseases.

Leptin: Why It's Working Against You

Leptin is your weight-loss hormone. Most people don't know they have such a thing. Magic happens when you discover how to make it work for you.

This appetite-suppressing, fat-burning hormone is the most powerful hormone that regulates your metabolism. When you've eaten enough, and your body fat has reached an adequate level, your fat cells release leptin. This hormone travels from your fat cells to your brain and tells it how much fat is available. As you store fat and gain weight, your fat cells send more leptin to the brain. The brain then slows down your eating (decreases appetite) and increases your metabolism (burns more fat), if this hormone is working correctly.

But when leptin levels are too high, this process stops working. This malfunction can make you eat more and gain weight.

Signs of leptin excess include

- Weight gain, hunger, and carbohydrate craving
- Slower metabolism
- Increased stress, irritability, and mood swings

Remember the angry fat cells from Chapter One? When these cells produce more and more leptin, you develop a syndrome called leptin resistance. In this scenario, no matter how much leptin is created in the fat cells, the brain's receptor sites do not "hear it"; they tune it out. When the brain does not hear the leptin, it thinks you are starving, so it sends your appetite into overdrive, slows your metabolism, and every bit of food gets stored on your belly!

How to Get Leptin Working for You

Make your leptin work for you by following the 7 Systems Plan. If you are doing this, your leptin is beginning to work again. These seven steps will speed up your progress even more:

1. Lower your intake of high-GI carbohydrates, fructose, and grains.
2. Stop overeating.
3. Use an FMD like the 5:2 Fast.
4. Decrease stress.
5. Get seven to eight hours of sleep.
6. Lower your insulin.
7. Lose weight.

As you do this, leptin will drop to a normal level, and this hormone will begin to work for you again.

Thyroid: Why It's Working Against You

Thyroid is your metabolism hormone. The thyroid gland is located under your Adam's apple and produces thyroid hormones. These master metabolism hormones control every function in your body. The thyroid produces T4 (inactive hormone) and T3 (active thyroid hormone). They affect your weight (fat burning), metabolism, mood, energy, body temperature, and the function of virtually every organ in your body.

Thyroid keeps your body running at the right speed. If it's set right, you have energy and burn calories fast. If it's set too low, you slow down and burn fewer calories. If you have low thyroid hormone, you may experience these symptoms:

- Weight gain
- Dry skin
- Hair loss
- Loss of the outer third of the eyebrow
- Low energy
- Feeling cold

Some experts believe that 50 million Americans may have low thyroid levels. Research shows that 1 in 5 women and 1 in 10 men are hypothyroid.[10]

What can compromise thyroid function?

- Toxins like cigarette smoke, mercury, and polychlorinated biphenyls (PCBs)
- Gluten sensitivity and intolerance
- Phytoestrogens from genetically modified, processed, non-organic soy
- Iodine deficiency
- Bromine from baked goods, plastics, and other sources
- Stress and elevated cortisol

How to Get Thyroid Working for You

Make your thyroid work for you by following the 7 Systems Plan. I also suggest following these steps:

1. A good multivitamin, fish oil, and vitamin D3 are a must. Iodine is no longer added to food or most salts, and deficiency can be a factor in thyroid function.
2. If your thyroid remains low, get a prescription for thyroid hormone. Synthroid and Levothyroxine (inactive T4 only) are the most prescribed. When possible, I think it is always better to use natural hormones rather than synthetic. I prefer natural thyroid prescriptions (like Armour, Westhroid, or Nature Thyroid), which contain T4 and T3 (the active form).
3. Go gluten free. If you have gluten intolerance, it can trigger an immune reaction. Your Defense System can mistake thyroid for gluten, causing it to come under attack.

Testosterone: Why It's Working Against You

Testosterone is your muscle and sex hormone. It is the key male hormone, manufactured in the testicles. Every cell in the male body has receptors for this hormone. It makes men grow muscles, have deep voices, and achieve erections. Women need testosterone too, in small amounts, and produce it in their ovaries.

Testosterone increases sexual interest, muscle mass, memory, and bone health. It also keeps skin from sagging, helps you lose weight, and provides you with an overall sense of well-being.

Signs of low testosterone include

- Weight gain
- Low sex drive
- Difficulty achieving erections
- Hair loss
- Fatigue
- Loss of muscle
- Mood changes

Testosterone levels often begin to drop at age 30 and plummet at age 50. Low testosterone can be caused by stress, toxins, lack of exercise, or too much body fat. When you have lots of body fat, your fat cells and testicles produce an enzyme called aromatase that converts testosterone into estrogen. Ever notice how obese males start to develop "man boobs"?

Low testosterone alters the way you metabolize fat and carbohydrates and has been linked to heart disease, hypertension, diabetes, and other diseases. If you are a male with low testosterone, you may die sooner than normal, and you certainly won't have as much fun.

How to Get Testosterone Working for You

Make your testosterone work for you by doing the following:

1. Make sure you are eating enough good fats, as they are used to make testosterone.
2. Avoid statin drugs that can block its production.

3. Follow the 7 Systems Plan, exercise correctly, and lose weight. I have had patients double their testosterone in 90 days by doing this alone.
4. Supplements can boost testosterone. The most effective that I recommend is Testro Balance.
5. For significantly low testosterone that does not respond to natural treatment, bioidentical hormone replacement therapy (BHRT) may be necessary. Two methods that seem to be the most successful are topical gels and weekly injections. As with all HRT, retesting is necessary until your level remains in the ideal zone.

Estrogen and Progesterone: Why They're Working Against You

Estrogen and progesterone are the two key female hormones. They balance each other out. This fact is important. One accumulates fat—the other burns it. One excites—the other calms. One retains fluid—the other eliminates it.

These hormones are responsible for the growth and development of female sexual characteristics and reproduction. Estrogen includes a group of hormones: estriol, estradiol, and estrone. Each has different functions throughout a woman's lifetime.

Excess estrogen in women causes breast tenderness, fluid retention, premenstrual syndrome, fibroids, and heavy menstrual bleeding. In a man, it causes loss of body hair, a beer belly, and man boobs. Excess estrogen will cause weight gain in both men and women. (If you need some extra proof, talk to a rancher who implants estrogen pellets in his steers to fatten them up.)

Progesterone plays a role in maintaining pregnancy, regulating the monthly cycle, and making other hormones (including DHEA, estrogen, testosterone, and cortisol). Progesterone deficiency may make it difficult to fall asleep.

Both estrogen and progesterone are produced in the testicles of men (in small amounts). Progesterone is used to make testosterone and helps to counteract the effects of estrogen.

Having an unhealthy lifestyle, poor diet, lack of exercise, micronutrient deficiencies, a weak Detox System, toxins, and many other things can throw these two hormones out of balance in your body. For women, the main thing that causes estrogen and progesterone levels to plummet is their age. As women enter menopause, low levels can affect their endocrine and nerve networks. In the endocrine networks, this means bleeding irregularities, vaginal dryness, hot flashes, and decreased sex drive. In the nerve networks, this means insomnia, nervousness, irritability, headaches, mood changes, and depression.

How to Get Estrogen and Progesterone Working for You

If you have high estrogen, eliminate the things that elevate it:

- Excess sugar, refined carbohydrates, and alcohol
- Antibiotic use or bad bacteria in your gut
- Constipation
- Too little fiber
- Environmental toxins that act like estrogen in your body (learn more in Chapter Seven)
- Lack of exercise

To address estrogen deficiency, follow these steps:

1. Besides following the 7 Systems Plan, take vitamin D, omega-3, black cohosh, and Estrovera. I have directed women to Estrovera for years to help them with menopausal symptoms. This natural product contains ERr 731 (an extract from rhubarb). It has been shown in clinical studies to decrease hot flashes by as much as 75% in just 12 weeks. This is similar to the benefit of hormone replacement therapy.[11]
2. If problems persist, get a lab hormone profile test and fix deficiencies using BHRT. When doing BHRT, you should never take estrogen without also correcting your

progesterone. The two must be balanced. Never take synthetic hormones. A much safer approach is to use bioidentical hormones.[12]

Nerves

In the early frontier days, telegraph wire was used to send messages between towns. If the wire was intact, communication could occur. In your body, messages travel through nerves that tell organs, muscles, and Systems what to do. Without this communication, your organs and System functions can be compromised.

Why Your Nerves Are Working Against You

Most of your nerves travel through the spinal column to get to their destination. This is why the spine is the most common place for nerve signal interference to occur. According to Matthew McCoy, "misalignments and/or abnormal motion [subluxations] of vertebral motion units may compromise neural integrity and may influence organ system function and general health...."[13]

If you have a forward head posture, an increased curve in your middle back, subluxations, or imbalances in your spine, you could be compromising the electrical flow through your nerves and impair their function.

How to Get Your Nerves Working for You

Chiropractic care can improve your nerve communication through spinal manipulation. Peter Rome weighs in: "Chiropractors are spinal and nerve specialist trained to detect subluxations in the spine (areas of potential nerve interference) and correct them. But the benefits of spinal manipulation go far beyond just spinal pain relief. A study reviewed more than 500 papers confirmed spinal manipulations beneficial effect on organ function, hormone function, immune function and cognitive issues."[14]

Even people without symptoms benefit from spinal manipulation. "Improved function can be objectively measured in asymptomatic individuals following chiropractic care in a number of body systems often by relatively non-invasive means. It is plausible that chiropractic care may be of benefit to every function of the body and have the potential for long-term, overall health benefit to those receiving chiropractic care."[15]

Heart rate variability (HRV) is a relatively new test used assess your health. Abnormal HRV is associated with dying sooner, depression, diabetes, impaired cognitive performance, and memory problems. In a study of 625 patients, the authors reported that "The chiropractic care group showed a significant improvement in HRV on both the single-visit and the 4-week visit groups, but not in the control group."[16]

As an added benefit, chiropractic care decreases surgery.[17] A study of 1,885 workers (174 of whom had lumbar spine surgery in the last three years) found that "approximately 42.7% of workers who first saw a surgeon had surgery, in contrast to only 1.5% of those who saw a chiropractor."[18]

How to Get Your Nervous System Working for You

1. Maintain proper posture.
2. Get regular spinal adjustments.

Neurotransmitters

Your brain has billions of nerve cells (neurons) that do not directly touch each other. Messages are passed from one neuron to the next by complex chemical messengers called neurotransmitters. If your nerves are the telegraph wire running between towns, your NTs are the people sitting in the telegraph office. They receive the messages and transfer them to the next wire so that the signals can continue along the nerve. All of your movements, thoughts, and feelings are the result of these NTs talking via electrical and chemical signals.

About 100 different neurotransmitters have been identified. They influence neurons in a specific part of your brain, affecting your mood, anxiety, hunger, and fear. They can either excite neurons or inhibit their activity. Norepinephrine, acetylcholine, and dopamine are excitatory neurotransmitters, while serotonin and GABA are calming.

We now know that 40 NTs and hormones are produced in your gut, so maintaining a healthy gut is vital for their correct function. In fact, more serotonin (the mood-elevating NT) and melatonin (the sleep NT) come from your gut than your brain. 95% of all the serotonin in your body is in the Digestive System. Your gut health is vital for both your physical and mental health.

Why Your Neurotransmitters (NTs) Are Working Against You

Stress, medications, and deficiencies in fundamental micronutrients can deplete your neurotransmitters. When these NTs are low, you will likely try to boost them in unhealthy ways. Sugar, alcohol, and some drugs can temporarily stimulate the release of more feel-good neurotransmitters and begin an unhealthy addiction.

Studies indicate that sugar may be one of the most addictive substances currently known. Some studies indicate sugar may be eight times more addictive than heroine!

94% of rats, when given a choice between sugar water and cocaine, chose sugar.[19]

When you eat sugar, it releases neurotransmitters that make you feel good temporarily and experience pleasure, so you want to eat more of it. Abnormally high stimulation of your receptors by sugar generates excessive reward signals in your brain that override the self-control mechanism (willpower). If you constantly stimulate these receptors, they downregulate (stop listening), so it takes more and more sugar to get the same pleasurable feeling. After only three weeks, these receptors can be downregulated so much that you are a sugar addict. The result is increased hunger, cravings, and overeating—not to get a buzz, but just to feel normal.

The trick to breaking food addiction is to stop eating feel-good foods. Temporary withdrawal is natural, but if you supply your body with the macronutrients and micronutrients it needs, your neurotransmitter levels will come back to normal and the receptors will begin to work again. Within 10 days of beginning the 7 Systems Plan, most of my patients' cravings and hunger decrease significantly, and they feel better.

Let's look at two key NTs that affect your weight: serotonin and dopamine.

Serotonin

Serotonin is the happiness neurotransmitter. It affects weight, mood, contentment, focus, concentration, and sleep. Signs of low serotonin include

- Weight gain
- Sugar craving
- Depression or worry
- Insomnia
- Low self-esteem

NeuroScience Lab research has shown that most people are low in NTs. 89% of the general public is low in serotonin, and 64% are low in norepinephrine. Women typically experience lower levels than men.

How to Get Serotonin Working for You

Make your serotonin work for you by doing the following:

1. Get more exercise.
2. Eat a healthy diet (the 7 Systems Plan).
3. Maintain quality relationships and talk to someone who cares.

4. Get enough sleep.

5. Cuddle with someone or take a warm bath.

6. Have more sex.

7. Take folate, omega-3 EPA and DHA, and probiotic supplements.

8. Consume dark chocolate (in limited amounts).

Dopamine

Dopamine is a gratification neurotransmitter. It helps regulate emotions, cognition, motivation, and feelings of pleasure. Signs of low dopamine include

- Weight gain
- Low energy
- Impatience
- Inattentiveness
- Impulsiveness
- Forgetfulness

Most drugs that people abuse—legal and illegal—are aimed at increasing dopamine release in your brain. Some drugs can increase NT release by up to 1,000%, making addiction probable. This high, like a sugar high, is followed by a low that causes the person to want another fix. It takes more and more of the drug to give the same effect, pushing them along the path to addiction.

Believe it or not, grains and starches are like drugs to your body. Potatoes and bread are comfort foods because they have a soothing, calming effect on your brain and trigger feelings of gratification. This is because they contain a compound called benzodiazepine. This same substance is found in the drugs Ativan, Xanax, and Valium. Cravings for comfort foods can be incredibly strong, even rivaling cravings for illegal drugs like heroin.

In a recent study,[20] two groups were fed either a milkshake with sugar (enters the bloodstream quickly) or a milkshake with starch (enters the bloodstream slowly). Both milkshakes had the same taste and calories. The subjects' brains were then scanned to see the effect.

In every case, the group with the fast-entering sugar had their brain's addiction and reward center (the nucleus encumbrance) light up like a Christmas tree within 30 minutes! This is the same area of the brain that lights up when heroin and other addictive drugs are consumed.

How to Get Dopamine Working for You

Make your dopamine work for you by doing the following:

1. Create healthy brain chemistry by having a healthy lifestyle. Dopamine is elevated by the opportunity to make a difference (service), high-protein diets, and vitamins including folate.
2. Avoid the wrong foods. Certain foods give a boost of dopamine that contributes to food addiction. Usually, these foods are a combination of sugary, fatty, and salty foods that are called hyper-palatables. These include potato chips, donuts, candy bars, and soft drinks. They can hijack the reward and pleasure system in your brain in the same way as illegal drugs.
3. Give it some time. Your desires will change, healthy food will taste better, and what you want to eat and how much you want to eat will change within a couple of weeks.

Addiction

Addiction and cravings can be caused by food and an imbalance of hormones and neurotransmitters. It is estimated that 1 in 12 people are food addicts. The majority are women. Food addiction is real, and it will prevent you from regaining your health.

Here are a few signs that you have an addiction to food:

1. You need to eat to feel normal.
2. You need carbohydrates in the morning.
3. You need more and more food to get the same good feeling.
4. You have symptoms if you do not have the food (headaches, fatigue, irritability, anxiety, sleep disturbance).

Overcoming food addiction is not only possible, but it's also imperative. If you need help, please join my online course for additional support. Here is a proven path to kick your cravings:

1. Acknowledge the craving and the foods you are addicted to.
2. Absolutely avoid the offending food. Draw a hard line between the things you can and cannot have.
3. Include protein with each meal and snack to encourage a slow, long rise in blood sugar.
4. Consume low-GI carbohydrates.
5. Avoid artificial sweeteners.
6. Use healthy foods to satisfy your sweet tooth, like a bowl of berries.
7. Balance your hormones and neurotransmitters.
8. Try an FMD for fast progress in breaking the addiction.

Quick Recap:

- Your lifestyle and diet have most likely weakened your Communication System. The core of fixing the Communication System should be following the 7 Systems Plan.
- Just as good food can balance your System, bad food can mess it up.
- Excessive hormones lead to receptor site resistance, which inhibits the hormones' effectiveness.
- A lack of the two major hormones, insulin and cortisol, will kill you. An excess will make you miserable.

- Correct the two major hormones first. Work on the others next if necessary.
- Leptin, thyroid, testosterone, estrogen, and progesterone are the minor hormones. Address these five if you need to. Each one needs to be at an ideal level for optimal health.
- Bioidentical hormone replacement therapy is sometimes needed and very helpful. If necessary, consult a BHRT provider. Get the proper lab work done so that you know your levels, and use only bioidentical hormones from a reputable compounding pharmacy. Use the minimum dose to fix your levels and resolve symptoms.
- Systems, organs, and cells depend on signals from the nervous system to function optimally.
- Proper spinal alignment allows for optimal nerve function.
- Neurotransmitter balance affects your brain function, mood, and weight.

Proven Steps to Fix Your Communication System:

(Check these off as you complete them. Join our free 7 Systems Plan Community for additional support and encouragement: 7SystemsPlan.com.)

☐ After fixing the two major hormones, fix the most serious minor one first and then move to the next. Undergo hormone testing if your problems do not resolve.

☐ Insulin and leptin are the hormones that are most likely to cause weight problems. Decrease bad carbohydrates and lose weight to lower them both.

☐ Schedule a spinal evaluation and maintain ideal nerve function.

☐ Optimize neurotransmitter levels the healthy way: Follow the 7 Systems Plan.

Supplements to Support Your Communication System

I use two products to support the Communication System. If you have diabetes or high insulin, you can use a functional food like the one Donna used to help her lose weight and eliminate her diabetes—Cardio-Metabolic. If you have estrogen regulation problems, try Dynamic Hormone Balance.

I provide more detail at 7SystemsPlan.com and in Appendix A, Part Five.

Communication System Lab Tests

Hormones

Simple At-Home Test: Pinch Test and Check Weight

- *Pinch:* Since high insulin makes you gain belly fat, pinch your belly. The more you have to pinch, the higher your insulin likely is. The ideal for men is half an inch. The ideal for women is one inch.
- *Scale:* Check your weight. If you are 20 pounds overweight, your insulin may have doubled. If you are 50 pounds overweight, your insulin may be 10 times higher than normal.

Tests for Insulin:

- *Fasting Insulin:* A fasting insulin test will tell you your level of insulin resistance. Your fasting insulin level should be less than 5 mcIU/mL. The higher it is, the more serious your problem. Any doctor who does lab testing can order this test for you.

Cortisol

- Your cortisol should be low when you wake, rise to a peak by mid-morning, and then slowly fall in the afternoon and evening. By using either a urine or saliva test that measures your cortisol at four different times during the day, you can see if you have a normal cortisol pattern, excess or insufficient cortisol, or more serious problems.

- Use the stress test questionnaire at 7SystemsPlan.com to see how much stress you have and which type you have.

Leptin

- A simple way to know if you have leptin resistance is to check your leptin level. Ideally, leptin should be less than 12 ng/ml. The higher it is, the more severe your issues are.
- Another way to estimate if you have high leptin is to pinch your belly. The more you have to pinch, the greater your chances are of having high leptin and leptin resistance syndrome.

Thyroid

- Check your temperature in the morning before you get out of bed. Do this each day for a week and record your temperature. If your temperature is below 97.2, you most likely have an underactive thyroid.
- A TSH (thyroid-stimulating hormone) test measures the amount of work your brain is asking your thyroid to do. The higher it is, the more likely you are hypothyroid. The old standard for TSH was that anything over 5 mU/L is abnormal, and many doctors still use this. In 2002, the normal range was changed so that anything greater than 3 is considered hypothyroid. Many doctors, myself included, believe that your TSH should be less than 2 to be in the healthy zone.
- Checking only your TSH level does not give you an accurate picture of how your thyroid is working. You should also have T3 (active thyroid hormone), T4 (inactive thyroid hormone), and reverse T3 (T3 going back to T4) checked to get the complete picture. (High reverse T3 means that your thyroid hormones are not working properly.)
- Other tests measure thyroid antibodies, including thyroid

peroxidase (TPO) and anti-thyroglobulin antibodies. Refer to 7SystemsPlan.com for more helpful information.

Testosterone

- Men of any age and females over age 40 should test their testosterone level.
- If you are a male, you can get an idea of whether or not you are low in testosterone by filling out the testosterone questionnaire at 7SystemsPlan.com.
- When you have your testosterone checked, make sure to test both your total testosterone and free testosterone. The free test measures the amount of testosterone circulating in the blood that is available to your body for immediate use. See 7SystemsPlan.com for more information on testing.
- Normal values for testosterone vary depending on which doctor or lab you talk to. Some say that total testosterone less than 200 ng/dL is abnormal. Others say less than 348 is abnormal. The bottom line is that higher testosterone makes you feel and act younger.

Estrogen and Progesterone

- I prefer to use urine or saliva testing for these two. Your test should measure all three estrogens (estriol, estradiol, and estrone) and progesterone. See 7SystemsPlan.com for more information.

Nerves

- Have a chiropractic spinal evaluation and posture analysis.
- Get a spinal X-ray.

Neurotransmitters

- Neurotransmitter imbalance can be detected by a lab test. Visit 7SystemsPlan.com for my recommendations.

6

The Defense System
Acute and Chronic Inflammation

Win the weight war with a good defense.

Startling Facts

- Antibiotic-resistant superbugs kill more than 23,000 per year.[1]
- Autoimmune diseases affect 8% of the population (approximately 24 million Americans) and are the third leading cause of death.[2]
- Silent inflammation affects up to 75% of all Americans.[3]

> *"By 2050 . . . antibiotic-resistant bacteria could kill an estimated 10 million people each year.* Shockingly, this would surpass even cancer."[4]
> —Julia Calderone

Let's imagine that your other five Systems have been working correctly up to this point:

- Your Structural System is supported with real food.
- Your Digestive System broke the food down into small nutrients.
- Your Delivery System picked up the nutrients and delivered them to the cells.
- Your Energy System (mitochondria) turned the nutrients into energy.
- Your Communication System ensured the proper function of each System with hormones, nerves, and neurotransmitters.

Now you must have a way to protect the Systems and your body. This is where the Defense System comes in.

A Brief Introduction to The Defense System

Your body is constantly under assault from enemies on the outside and inside. Fortunately, you have a whole army in reserve waiting for the signal to attack these foreign invaders and heal the injured tissue. This army includes mast cells, histamines, cytokines, inflammatory molecules, macrophages, neutrophils, and lymphocytes. Without your Defense System to thwart off hostile invaders, you would die in a few days.

The key to proper Defense System function, like most things in life, is balance. If the Defense System is underactive, you're likely to get colds, ear infections, bronchitis, and other infections. If this System is overactive, you are more susceptible to allergies, asthma, food sensitivities, and autoimmune disease.

A malfunction in any of the seven Systems—including your Defense System—can sabotage weight-loss efforts. If you can get this System to work for you, it will do a fantastic job at defending your body from infection, inflammation, and deadly diseases. Besides these benefits, you'll also discover that weight loss is much easier.

7 Signs That Your Defense System Is Working Against You:

1. Weight gain
2. Frequent colds or flu
3. Chronic pain, joint pain with exercise, swollen joints, and inflammation
4. Skin problems
5. Infections (sinus, urinary tract, athlete's foot)
6. Periodontal disease
7. Frequent anti-inflammatory or antibiotic use

Meet Sharon

Several years ago, after teaching a class on the Defense System, I got a call from a lady living in another state. A patient who was in my class had given my number to her and asked her to call me. Her name was Sharon.

Sharon had developed severe pain and swelling in her joints. I could hear the concern in her voice. She explained in a shaky tone that she had so much pain, she had to sleep in a chair. I knew this was only compounding her problems. How much sleep can you get while sitting in a chair? The pain in her feet was so bad that she could not wear shoes. Understandably, walking was difficult. Her increasing weight made matters worse.

She had also developed pain in her hands, making it difficult to use her computer mouse. She got sick frequently. Sharon feared losing her job as an accountant.

Sharon's medical doctor had run some tests and sent her to a rheumatologist for a further workup. The rheumatologist diagnosed her with rheumatoid arthritis. This incurable, disabling autoimmune disease is caused by an overactive Defense System attacking the joints. When she went in for the report, she was prescribed a powerful drug to suppress her Defense System.

Once she got home, she went online and looked at the side effects of this drug. Immediately, she felt discouraged. On her return visit to the rheumatologist, she asked him, "Can I help this problem by changing my lifestyle?" His prompt reply was, "No, you must take the drug."

After hearing her history, I concluded that we should focus our initial treatment on her Defense System. It was working against her. I gave her a list of additional lab tests, which included evaluating her inflammation level, liver function, and vitamin D.

Vitamin D deficiency is often connected with autoimmune diseases and is a significant factor in rheumatoid arthritis. The lab test confirmed the battle that was going on inside her. Her vitamin D level was 6 ng/ml; it should have been over 50. Her other tests showed high inflammation and signs of fatty liver disease.

Sharon followed the 7 Systems Plan and implemented the information in this chapter. Her progress was slow but consistent, and in six months, all signs of rheumatoid arthritis had disappeared. She was not only wearing shoes again, but she was jogging in those shoes. She hadn't done that in years. The pain in her hands disappeared, and she lost 65 pounds. Her Defense System was no longer attacking her body. Instead, it was working for her.

Sharon's thank you note captured her gratitude. She wrote, "I'm convinced you can make a difference in your health by the choices you make. Thank you, Dr. Pat, I am so grateful for your guidance!"

Why Your Defense System Is Working Against You

When the Defense System is activated, it sets an inflammatory process in motion. Acute inflammation is the Defense System's response to localized injury or attack. Think of it as a fire that destroys the enemy and begins the healing process.

Here's a quick example of an injury and your body's response.

Acute Inflammation: The Fire Within

Imagine getting a splinter of wood in your finger. As the wood breaks the skin, cells are destroyed and your skin barrier is damaged, allowing bacteria to get into the body. You are alerted to this threat by the pain from sensory nerves in your finger. Your Defense System is now activated, and the mast cells (white blood cells) at the site release histamines and cytokines to send a signal for help throughout the body. This distress call activates the production of inflammatory molecules. They turn on the inflammation process (fire) in your body to help correct the problem.

The blood vessels allow other immune cells into the injured area (causing swelling) to defend against foreign material. The fire continues as macrophages start attacking the bacteria and damaged cells, releasing defensive chemicals. Your body's neutrophils are drawn to the wound and begin to engulf and destroy the bacteria and damaged tissue. Lymphocytes also join the battle and help in the cleanup. Platelets and other substances form clots to close the wound and stop the bleeding.

As the bacteria and damaged tissue are eliminated, cells from your body signal that the fire is no longer needed, and the process ends. This resolution is critical. The complicated process of defense, acute inflammation, and resolution is necessary for your survival.

Chronic Inflammation: The Fire Does Not Go Out

For many people today, the feverish scenario described above never stops. The Defense System does not shut down. When acute inflammation becomes chronic, your Defense System begins to work against you. It is believed that chronic inflammation is the strongest predictor of disease development. It is linked to heart disease, cancer, Alzheimer's disease, and many more illnesses.

Unfortunately, foreign invaders aren't the only ones that can trigger this inflammatory response in your body. The average American lifestyle (diet high in sugar and saturated fat, vitamin deficiencies, lack of exercise, excess body fat, faulty GI tract, toxins, high blood pressure, high insulin, stress, periodontal disease, some drugs) makes it easier for your body to get stuck in this chronically inflamed state.

It is crucial to address the cause and fix the System by providing the nutrients necessary to resolve inflammation. If your Defense System is not working correctly, you may experience weight gain, chronic disease at a young age, and even an early death. You must give your body what it needs to put out the fire.

Autoimmune Diseases

When the Defense System is active for too long, it can start attacking the body. This is known as autoimmune disease, which affects 8% of the population—approximately 24 million Americans. 80% of those affected are women. It is estimated that less than one-third of those who have it are diagnosed, and the rates are increasing dramatically.[5]

Autoimmune diseases are now the third leading cause of morbidity and mortality (after heart disease and cancer). There are over 80 different types. The more common ones are rheumatoid arthritis, lupus, Graves' disease, psoriasis, multiple sclerosis, Crohn's disease, colitis, type 1 diabetes, and celiac disease.

While these conditions can have a genetic component, we now suspect that 70% of the cause involves environment, diet, and lifestyle. Many doctors do not know that the Defense System can be fixed, so they consider autoimmune diseases incurable. Healthcare costs for autoimmune diseases are two times higher than cancer treatment.

How to Get Your Defense System Working for You

Step 1: Eliminate Defense System problems caused by diet.

A lack of essential macronutrients and micronutrients can compromise your Defense System. You may also have problems if you overconsume unhealthy macronutrients. Recent studies have shown that high consumption of sugar and bad fats can cause post-meal inflammation.[6] If this happens frequently, it increases your chances of developing diabetes and cardiovascular diseases.

Restricting calories has a powerful effect on lowering inflammation, but simply eating *less* isn't the solution. You need to eat *better* too.

The solution is to restrict calories properly and eat an anti-inflammatory diet (the 7 Systems Plan). Historically, diets were naturally anti-inflammatory. They used to be high in fruits and vegetables and rarely included sugar. Meats were limited to lean game, wildfowl, and fish. Healthy eggs supplied additional protein. As a result, there were few degenerative inflammatory diseases like arthritis, diabetes, heart disease, and Alzheimer's disease.

Today, our diets are based on inflammatory foods like grains, milk, sugar, grain and seed oils, saturated fats, and alcohol. At the same time, the intake of fruits, vegetables, and legumes has decreased.

Adopting an anti-inflammatory diet through the 7 Systems Plan seems to be the most effective strategy for turning off chronic inflammation.

Step 2: Eliminate Defense System problems caused by an unhealthy Digestive System.

Your intestinal health is of paramount importance to your Defense System. 70% of your Defense System tissue surrounds your Digestive System. This defense tissue can help upregulate your entire body's Defense System, making it more active when needed or less active when not needed. Without a healthy intestinal tract, your Defense System can get stuck in a hyperactive state, resulting in chronic inflammation.

If you don't chew your food enough or have acid or enzyme deficiencies, your food may not break down enough as it goes through your Digestive System. This can damage the intestinal tract and trigger a defense response. Your body sees these undigested molecules as foreign invaders and attacks them, causing tissue damage. When this happens, the tight junctions between cells in the intestines can widen, allowing material to "leak" into the body. Leaky gut syndrome can activate the production of inflammatory defense molecules that lead to chronic inflammation.

To repair a leaky gut, I use a low-allergen functional food called Dynamic Detox (see Chapter Two). It contains vital micronutrients that turn off these inflammatory signals and heal the gut tissue. Learn more about this product at 7SystemsPlan.com.

Step 3: Eliminate Defense System problems caused by bad bacteria.

In 1928, medicine was forever changed by the discovery of penicillin—the first antibiotic. Suddenly, we held a lot of power over some of the deadliest diseases known to humankind. Infections from cuts and cases of strep throat used to kill people. But thanks to the availability of antibiotics, these illnesses no longer take lives.

However, like many good things, antibiotics came with a price tag. Doctors overprescribed them, and people began to self-treat with them. More than one-third of the patients who visit clinics in the U.S. are inappropriately prescribed these "miracle drugs," often for symptoms caused by viruses that antibiotics cannot even kill.[7]

Because of overuse and inappropriate use (including the low-dose antibiotics that are used in agriculture), we have created resistant bacteria called superbugs. The bacteria we set out to destroy are now mutating, exchanging genetic material, and multiplying. Antibiotic-resistant bacteria are hard to kill and are associated with 23,000 deaths annually in the United States.[8]

Bad bacteria, yeast, parasites, and a lack of good bacteria can damage your intestines, triggering a defense response. When the bad bacteria outnumber the good bacteria, you absorb toxins that trigger inflammation. Gut microbial imbalances are associated with gastritis, irritable bowel syndrome, inflammatory bowel disease, food allergies, skin problems, ulcers, autoimmune diseases, and yeast infections.

You need good bacteria, and not just in your gut. Different types of bacteria colonize your arms, hands, mouth, and every other part of your body. These friends help keep you healthy. Using antibacterial soap or mouthwash can eliminate these helpful bacteria and decrease the protection they provide.

Probiotics help, but when taking a probiotic, make sure your supplement is GMP certified, contains the kind of bacteria you need, has been proven to survive stomach acid, and is the right potency for you. If in doubt, order a test to check your

GI bacteria. This test will tell you the amount of good and bad bacteria in your GI tract. Again, refer to 7SystemsPlan.com for more help.

Step 4: Eliminate Defense System problems caused by key nutrient deficiencies.

Deficiencies in micronutrients can compromise your body's ability to turn on your Defense System when needed. Deficiencies can also keep your System from turning off.

Of all the micronutrients you need to thrive, vitamin D3 is at the top of the list. It seems to have the ability to balance our Defense System and keep it from under- or over-functioning. It's important to keep your vitamin D3 blood levels between 50 and 70 ng/ml. The higher end would be better if you have an autoimmune disease.

Turmeric is a plant with extraordinary anti-inflammatory properties. It can be ingested in many ways. My favorite is a functional food called Dynamic Inflam-Eze (see Appendix A, Part Five). It contains the form of curcumin (a component of turmeric) that is more biologically active than others, along with additional anti-inflammatory micronutrients. I take one scoop of this daily to prevent inflammation in my own body.

Vitamin C, folate, zinc, phytonutrients, and some amino acids are also essential for the Defense System's proper function.

Step 5: Eliminate Defense System problems caused by fatty acid imbalance.

It is estimated that 75% of all Americans have what is known as silent inflammation.[9] It is the underlying factor in everything from Alzheimer's to weight problems. This is due in part to the standard American diet being high in omega-6 and low in omega-3. These fatty acids control inflammation—one turns it on, and the other turns it off.

Omega-6 is proinflammatory. It's found in corn, safflower, cottonseed, and soybean oils; grains; and packaged foods. Excessive omega-6 promotes excess inflammation that goes beyond the normal healing process and promotes disease. It can lead to arthritis, headaches, osteoporosis, asthma, menstrual cramps, cancer, colitis, heart disease, and thrombus stroke.

Omega-3	Omega-6
Decreases clotting	Increases clotting
Dilates arteries	Constricts arteries
Anti-inflammatory	Proinflammatory
Decreases cancer risk	Increases cancer risk
Enhances immune system	Suppresses immune system

Omega-3 is anti-inflammatory. It's found in wild-caught fish, fish oil, nuts, wild game, grass-fed animals, green vegetables, flaxseed, and chia seeds. When you increase the amount of omega-3 in your diet, it displaces inflammatory compounds in your body and blocks inflammation.

If you do not have enough omega-3 fatty acids in your blood, it will be hard to stop inflammation once it has begun. The average American diet contains only 0.12 grams of this good fatty acid per day. To resolve inflammation, you need to take in at least two to six grams of omega-3 per day.

Omega-6 to Omega-3 Ratio of Foods	
Green vegetables	1:1
Fresh fish	1:1
Grass-fed meat	2.5:1 (varies)
Wild game	2.5:1 (varies)
Fruits	3:1

Omega-6 to Omega-3 Ratio of Foods	
Sweet potatoes	4:1
Nuts	5:1 or worse
Grain-fed meat	5:1 or worse
Grain-fed chicken (white)	15:1
Grain-fed chicken (dark)	17:1 (varies)
Grains (cereal, bread, pasta)	20:1 (varies)
Potato chips	60:1
Grain and vegetable oils	70–100:1

As you can see from the table, if you eat processed foods or consume harmful oils, it is impossible to maintain the ideal ratio of omega-6 to omega-3 in your diet (2:1). A fatty acid balance is essential for healthy cell membranes and blood vessel lining (see Chapter Three).

Consuming healthy fatty acids can also help you lose weight. Six weeks of increased omega-3 (EPA and DHA) intake significantly improves lean mass and decreases fat mass in healthy adults.[10]

If you have significant inflammatory problems, I suggest a product called PRM Resolve (see Appendix A, Part Five). Initial evidence shows that it may be a powerful supplement for those suffering from inflammatory conditions.[11],[12],[13]

Step 6: Eliminate Defense System problems caused by a lack of sleep.

We cannot address your Defense System without talking about sleep. Your Defense System can be severely compromised by lack of sleep because that's when your body repairs itself. Sleep deprivation moves your body into a chronically inflamed state by increasing your white blood cell levels. It makes you gain weight, catch more colds, and it impairs your body's insulin function.

Unfortunately, many people do not get enough sleep. According to the National Sleep Foundation, 20% of Americans sleep fewer than five hours per night. Other studies show this figure may be as high as 40%. Compared to those who get at least seven hours of sleep, people who sleep fewer than six hours per night quadruple their risk of catching a cold.[14]

Surprisingly, sleeping too much may be an even bigger problem. In one study, subjects with too little sleep weighed about 4.5 pounds more than the normal sleepers while those who slept too long weighed nearly 9 pounds more.[15]

Over 300 studies suggest that to protect your health, you need to make sure that you get adequate sleep. Seven to nine hours seems to be the magic zone. In a recent study, those who slept fewer than seven hours or more than nine hours per night weighed more than those who slept the recommended seven to nine hours.[16]

In another study, researchers reviewed data from 11 sleep studies involving more than 170 people. They found that limited sleep (typically about four hours a night) caused subjects to eat more the next day than when they ate after a full night's rest. On average, the sleep deprived ate 385 extra calories the next day, including more fat and less protein.[17]

Sleeping pills are not the answer. Studies show that people who take sleeping pills are not only at higher risk for certain cancers, they are also four times more likely to die than those who do not take them.[18]

If you are not getting a good night's sleep, review the sleep suggestions at 7SystemsPlan.com. If you continue to have problems, I suggest a natural sleep supplement called GoodNight (see Appendix A, Part Five). It includes melatonin, herbs, and minerals that promote healthy sleep and muscle relaxation.

Step 7: Be aware of Defense System problems caused by gluten and food allergies/sensitivities.

If you have Defense System problems or an autoimmune disease, you should look into the possibility that gluten intolerance or sensitivity could be the cause.

Up to 18 million Americans lack the enzymes needed to break down the gluten in wheat, rye, barley, and other grains.[19] Because they can't break it down, their bodies attack it as a foreign material. This defense reaction can harm your intestinal lining and trigger chronic inflammation. If left untreated, this damages your villi (the small, thumb-like structures lining your intestinal tract), hindering the absorption of nutrients. This condition is known as celiac disease.

Some people do not have an intolerance to gluten, just a sensitivity to it. Their reaction might not be as severe, but they still can't process gluten correctly.

Everyone with GI problems, skin problems, headaches, or an autoimmune disease should undergo a gluten sensitively test or simply remove gluten from their diet.

A few years ago, a mother brought her 10-year-old son into my clinic. He'd had a rash on his abdomen since birth. No treatment had resolved the rash. I suggested that she put him on a gluten-free diet to see if that might be the cause of his skin condition. In one month, the 10-year rash was gone!

If you are gluten intolerant or even sensitive, it will be very challenging for you to fix your Defense System and get healthy if you do not remove all sources of gluten from your diet.

Food Allergies and Sensitivities

If you want to know the food you are allergic to, it is probably the food that you crave the most. There is a very good chance that you are intolerant or sensitive to some food that you eat every day. When we expose our bodies to the same thing over and over, we're more likely to develop an intolerance. Inflammation caused by eating these foods is linked to a wide variety of chronic health problems.

There are two main categories of food allergies. Immunoglobulin E (IgE) causes severe symptoms within minutes or hours. Think of a peanut allergy—hives, swollen mouth, vomiting, and even death. The second is Immunoglobulin G (IgG), which is more delayed and causes milder symptoms—IBS, headaches, itchy skin, muscle stiffness, depression, fatigue, etc.

Some food allergies can be detected by the elimination diet. With this diet, you remove all potentially offending foods for 10 days and then add them back slowly, making sure to observe any signs or symptoms. (You can find details on the elimination diet at 7SystemsPlan.com.) This can be a little tricky because the symptoms are not always immediate, and sometimes the symptoms that do appear are not related to the GI tract. If you have a stuffy nose, itchy skin, or a cough after eating certain foods, you should consider the possibility that you have an allergy to that food.

The best way to know if you have food allergies is to have a food allergy test panel (Alcat). With a couple of tubes of your blood, the lab can check your body's reactions to 100+ foods, which are rated by severity—mild, moderate, or severe. This will give you and your physician the information you need to help you get on a healthy eating plan.

See a list of more tests at the end of the chapter.

Quick Recap:

- Your body uses acute inflammation to protect, heal, and repair itself.
- Both phases of inflammation—initiation and resolution—must work correctly.
- Chronic inflammation (lack of resolution) results in your Defense System working against you.
- Your diet and lifestyle can disrupt your Defense System and cause chronic inflammation.
- Eating an anti-inflammatory diet—found within the 7 Systems Plan—can support your Defense System.
- Underactive and overactive defense functions are both unhealthy.

- An overactive Defense System can lead to autoimmune diseases.
- Your gut health and good bacteria are of paramount importance to proper Defense System function.
- Eating the right macronutrients and micronutrients supports your Defense System.
- The ideal ratio of omega-6 to omega-3 (2:1) controls inflammation.
- Inadequate sleep can impair your Defense System.

Proven Steps to Fix Your Defense System:

(Check these off as you complete them. Join our free 7 Systems Plan Community for additional support and encouragement: 7SystemsPlan.com.)

☐ Take a good GMP certified probiotic.

☐ Increase your consumption of omega-3 and decrease omega-6 fat.

☐ Identify your primary defense problem and eliminate it.

Supplements to Support Your Defense System

In addition to adding probiotics, Sharon used two very helpful functional food products to support her Defense System.

The first is the functional food Dynamic Inflam-Eze, which helps support healthy inflammatory markers and gut function.

The second is Dynamic GI Restore. This product is designed to provide gastrointestinal nutritional support. The formula is uniquely designed to aid in promoting the growth of beneficial bacteria by including prebiotic nutrients combined with readily digestible macronutrients. It offers nutritional support for the management of compromised gut function, where most Defense System problems start.

See Appendix A, Part Five, for more supplement recommendations.

Defense System Lab Tests

Simple At-Home Test: Joint and Skin Test

Look at your hands: Enlarged joints can be a sign of Defense Systems malfunction.

Look at your skin: Eczema, psoriasis, and rashes can all be a sign of Defense System malfunction.

The hs-CRP Test

High-sensitivity C-reactive protein (hs-CRP) is produced in the liver in response to inflammation and provides an accurate indication of your inflammation level. A high hs-CRP level is a risk factor for disease and illness. Less than 1 mg/dL is a good level.

Sedimentation Rate

Sedimentation rate, or erythrocyte sedimentation rate (ESR), is another blood test that can reveal the amount of inflammation in your body. The higher the number, the more inflammation you have.

These are normal values:
    Men: 0-15 millimeters
    Women: 0-20 millimeters

Omega-6 to Omega-3 Ratio

A healthy ratio of inflammatory omega-6 and anti-inflammatory omega-3 is 2:1. This test measures your cell content for omega-3, omega-6, saturated fat, trans fat, and carbohydrate overconsumption.

The blood test is combined with a 20-minute online cognitive function test that shows how your fatty acid levels affect your focus/attention, memory, processing speed, cognitive flexibility, and risk for Alzheimer's disease. See 7SystemsPlan.com for information on a home test kit for the BrainSpan test.

Gluten

A comprehensive and accurate way to evaluate your gluten problems is to get a Cyrex Lab Array 3 test. This test will pick up gluten sensitivity that other methods won't find. Learn more at 7SystemsPlan.com.

Alcat

The standard method of checking for food allergies is measuring IgG, but there are potential problems with this approach. Alcat does the test differently. They measure your white blood cells' reaction to each food and grade it as normal, mild, moderate, or severe. Learn more at 7SystemsPlan.com.

7

The Detox System
Liver, Kidney, Colon, Lungs, and Skin

It's time to clean house.

Startling Facts

- Americans today have 30,000 to 50,000 chemicals in their bodies that their grandparents did not have. Many of these chemicals have been linked to the rapidly rising incidence of chronic childhood diseases.[1]
- Atrazine is a common herbicide that is present in 94% of drinking water tested by the USDA. Studies have linked atrazine exposure to impaired sexual development, some cancers, congenital disabilities, and infertility.[2]
- Other endocrine-disrupting chemicals such as BPA (in plastics) have been associated with impaired brain

development, lower IQs, infertility, congenital disabilities, obesity, diabetes, and endometriosis.[3]

"If your fish is sick because of a toxic fish tank, do you give it medicine for the symptoms or clean the fish tank?"
—Jason Vale, *Super Juice Me! Documentary*

Let's imagine that your other six Systems have been working correctly up to this point:

- Your Structural System is supported with real food.
- Your Digestive System broke the food down into small nutrients.
- Your Delivery System picked up the nutrients and delivered them to the cells.
- Your Energy System (mitochondria) turned the nutrients into energy.
- Your Communication System ensured the proper function of each System with hormones, nerves, and neurotransmitters.
- Your Defense System is on guard protecting your body.

With all of this work being done, cleanup has to take place. That is where your Detox System comes in.

A Brief Introduction to The Detox System

In the age we live in, we are exposed to more toxins than any previous generation. These toxins come in the form of chemicals, metals, medications, and toxins formed inside our bodies.

Think of your Detox System as a cleaning crew. It gets rid of toxins that have gotten into your body from the outside and eliminates waste and harmful material produced by your Systems. There are five primary workers on this cleaning crew:

1. Liver
2. Kidneys

3. Colon
4. Lungs
5. Skin

Each member of the crew must work effectively, or your weight will go up and your health will go down.

Most people think of a detox or cleansing program as a way to purge their System of the poor food they have eaten. Some just detox to lose weight.

While it certainly helps with weight loss, cleansing or detoxing benefits your entire body. Supporting your Detox System will help you lose weight (Structural System) and re-establish good bacteria in your gut (Digestive System). It will help deliver the nutrients you eat to your cells (Delivery System) and get your hormones (Communication System) to work for you again. You will have more energy (Energy System) and naturally heal faster (Defense System). I hope you are beginning to see how each System impacts the function of the other Systems and the importance of having them all function optimally.

7 Signs That Your Detox System Is Working Against You:

1. Weight gain
2. Brain fog or ringing in the ears
3. Muscle pain
4. Tingling in the hands or feet
5. Skin problems
6. Decreased energy
7. Sensitivity to food, medications, fragrances, alcohol, MSG, cigarette smoke, smog, or caffeine

Meet Beth

A woman named Beth came into my office to ask for help with her back pain. After learning her medical history, I knew there was more going on than problems with her Structural System. She explained that over the last year she had seen several specialists trying to get to the root of her problem but with no results.

She had constant pain all over her body, and it was significant enough that she could not walk without assistance. She had no energy, felt exhausted all the time, and was overweight. Work was extremely difficult for her, and she had been forced to quit her job six months before.

I suspected a problem with her Detox System. I asked Beth about exposure to toxins, but she said she had none. Further questioning revealed that her job cleaning the bank for the last 10 years had required the use of many cleaning solvents, and she had not used gloves.

Physical examination revealed tenderness under the right ribs and significant abdominal fat. Lab tests showed elevated liver enzymes (fatty liver), low salivary pH, obesity, high LDL cholesterol and GGT (toxicity), and low vitamin D. I suggested that we begin a detox program aimed at restoring normal function to her Detox System.

Although I didn't know it at the time, Beth wasn't too pleased with my suggestion. Months later, she told me about her first impressions: "You arrogant doctor! I have been to all these specialists, and you are going to make me feel better by detoxifying me? I'll show you. You do not know what you're talking about. I will do it, and it will not work."

The first few days of Beth's program were difficult, but she persisted. Within a week, her pain had dramatically decreased and her energy increased. By the time she completed the detox program, she labeled her own progress as "remarkable."

She was able to move without pain and before long returned to work.

She stuck with the 7 Systems Plan, and over the next few months she lost 60 pounds, had her lab tests return to normal, and got the rest of her Systems working correctly. She is now a strong advocate for fixing your Systems to restore your health.

It does seem remarkable that toxins could cause such severe symptoms, but it's true. And if you are going to lose weight, you must support this System.

A doctor instructing a patient to lose weight without addressing their Detox System should be considered malpractice. Most toxins in your body end up stored in your fat. When you empty these fat cells, you can release a flood of toxins into your body. The good news is that if you are following the steps in this book, you have already begun to detox and support your Detox System.

Why Toxins Are Working Against You

When I was a child, I would walk into the small, local general store with my dad. The owner would welcome us by name and take care of us. That is how handling toxins used to be for our bodies—there weren't many, and they were easy to handle.

Today, the toxins you are exposed to are like shoppers at a Walmart on Black Friday. When the door opens, they pour in. It's overwhelming. Most people come into contact with a plethora of toxins every day. It is impossible to process and eliminate all the toxins because there are so many. They often accumulate in your fat and continue to poison you over time.

Obesity and diabetes are only two of the many health problems associated with exposure to toxins. I believe most chronic diseases have their root in two major problems: toxicity and deficiencies of the nutrients needed to detox. If you are going to stay healthy and lose weight, it is imperative that your Detox System function well.

You eliminate many toxins through your urine, bowel movements, breathing, and sweat. Consider the following facts:

- If you do not take in enough water (half of your body weight in ounces per day), you impair toxin elimination from your kidneys.
- If you are constipated (not having at least one bowel moment per day), you reabsorb toxins in your colon.

- If you breathe polluted air or breathe incorrectly (through your mouth, too shallowly, or too deeply), you impair detox through your lungs.
- If your liver is not working well because of vitamin deficiencies or fatty liver disease, fat-soluble toxins will not be converted into forms that can be eliminated by your liver.
- If you do not sweat or exercise hard enough to perspire, you impair detox through your skin.

All of the toxins you are exposed to fit into one of two categories:

1. Toxins you take in
2. Toxins formed inside your body

Toxins in both categories have increased tremendously in the last 50 years. Every year, a total of 9.5 trillion pounds of chemicals are manufactured or imported into the United States. This translates into 30,000 pounds per American! So where do all these chemicals go? They go into food production, building materials, household products, personal care items, furniture, clothing, etc., but eventually, many of them go into you.

The water, soil, and air are contaminated by chemical emissions and runoff in greater amounts than ever before. Genetically engineered seeds require farmers to use more chemicals than they have ever used. Over one billion pounds of pesticides are used in America each year.

In the CDC's fourth national report on human exposure to environmental chemicals, they tested for 212 toxic chemicals and found all of them in the blood and urine of most test subjects.[4]

A study by Environmental Working Group in 2005 found that even unborn babies are being exposed to many of these toxic chemicals. 287 chemicals were detected in the umbilical cord blood of newborns. Almost all of these chemicals were known to cause cancer in humans or animals. Many were toxic to the brain and nerves, and some were known to cause congenital disabilities or abnormal development.[5]

Toxins can make you gain weight. Recent evidence shows that a variety of environmental endocrine disrupting chemicals (obesogens) increase fat cell formation and chances of obesity. These toxins make gaining weight easier. Chemicals like PCB, polybrominated diphenyl ethers, and perfluoro-compounds can disrupt hormonal signaling and cause you to gain weight. Exposure to Bisphenol A (BPA) is also is linked to obesity.[6]

BPA and phthalates are industrial chemicals used to make plastics more flexible and resilient. They are known as the "everywhere chemicals" and are in disposable water bottles, shower curtains, food packaging, vinyl flooring, household cleaners, cosmetics, personal care products, and even food. These endocrine disruptors are similar in structure to natural sex hormones such as estrogen and interfere with their function. Constant exposure can cause many problems:

- Feminization in men[7]
- Lower IQs in children[8]
- Increased PCOS
- Miscarriages
- Autism
- Asthma
- And many other health problems[9]

If you google obesogens, you will find hundreds of articles connecting common toxins to the obesity epidemic. Remember, most people are exposed to these toxins on a daily basis. You must decrease your exposure and increase your body's ability to eliminate them if you want to experience amazing health transformations and lasting weight loss.

Toxic Medication

In a study published in *JAMA: The Journal of the American Medical Association*, researchers found that 60% of all Americans take prescription drugs. Americans are about 5% of the world's population and consume 75% of the world's prescriptions.

Most people don't know that it is the Detox System's job to remove medications from the body. The problem is that we all eliminate drugs from our bodies differently, and some people are born with a weaker Detox System. If you are not able to detox, prescription drugs can damage your body and health. When you combine drugs, it becomes even harder for your body to process and remove them from your body. No wonder about 7% of all hospitalized patients are admitted because of adverse drug reactions![10]

Many prescription drugs cause weight gain, including common drugs used for diabetes, high blood pressure, and depression. There is a myth that over-the-counter medications are safe and do not need to be taken with caution. NSAIDs (over-the-counter pain medications) cause 16,500 deaths per year and are the 15th leading cause of death in America. Over 107,000 people are hospitalized annually due to its intestinal side effects alone.[11]

I encourage my patients to fix their Systems so that they do not need medication. Using the 7 Systems Plan, my patients work with their family doctor (as you should) to *safely* stop taking their medication for blood pressure, diabetes, acid reflux, cholesterol, and many more issues.

Dave is one example. When he came to my office, he was taking 43 prescription pills per day! Four months later, he was down to four pills.

Alice was on eight prescriptions when she came to see me. A few months later, her family doctor took her off all of them.

The reductions in Alice's and Dave's prescriptions were a result of fixing their Systems. Although it may sound unbelievable, you can reverse diseases like hypertension, hyperlipidemia, heart disease, diabetes, and even dementia. You can almost always get your body to the point where it does not need medication. Just fix your Systems, and work with your doctor.

Toxic Metals

Toxic metals are metals that your body does not require to function, and they are dangerous. Lead and mercury are two examples. Today, we all have metal toxins in our bodies that affect our weight and health.

Maybe you have heard the tragic story of lead in the drinking water of Flint, Michigan. Corrosive lead pipes in the city water system caused lead contamination in many homes, leading to serious health consequences. This story was reported, but thousands of incidents like this are never reported.

The Natural Resources Defense Council reports that anywhere from 15 million to 22 million Americans drink water that comes through lead pipes. Lead—even in tiny amounts—can damage intelligence and hearing and cause behavioral problems, especially in children.

Mercury is even more toxic than lead and can enter your body from dental amalgams, vaccinations, the fish you eat, the air you breathe, and the water you drink. This toxin can damage your body's nervous, cardiovascular, endocrine, and immune systems.

Toxic metals also inhibit your thyroid function. Metals can impair T4 (inactive form) to T3 (active form) conversion. This puts an invisible force field around your body fat so that it becomes difficult to lose weight.

Toxic Material Formed in Your Body

Toxins are a by-product of many normal processes within your body. They form when hormones are broken down, food is metabolized, energy is produced, and tissues are repaired. These toxins are a part of life, and your body has a way to deal with them—if your Detox System is healthy.

In your Digestive System, good bacteria help prevent toxins from entering your body. Conversely, bad bacteria can damage the protective lining of your gut and also produce toxins. Imbalances in your Communication System can burden your Detox System. Chronic inflammation from a compromised Defense System adds to the toxicity.

You get the picture—each of your Systems affects the health and proper function of the others.

How to Get Your Detox System Working for You

Turn your Detox System from an enemy into an ally by limiting your exposure to toxins.

How to Limit Your Exposure to Toxins:

- Eat mostly fresh, real, whole foods.
- Avoid high-mercury fish and eat low-mercury fish instead (see a detailed list in Appendix A, Part One).
- Increase elimination of toxic metals by eating sulfur-rich eggs, onions, garlic, leeks, and asparagus.
- Be cautious of silver (mercury) dental fillings.
- Avoid drinking water from lead plumbing.
- Avoid processed and packaged foods (especially from cans), which are a common source of BPA and phthalates.
- Avoid plastic wraps and never microwave food or beverages in plastic or Styrofoam. Store your food in glass, stainless steel, and wax paper.
- Replace your vinyl shower curtain with a fabric one.
- Limit your handling of cash register receipts, which can contain BPA.
- Avoid plastics in every form.
- Avoid nonstick and aluminum cookware. Use stainless steel, cast iron, glass, and enamel cookware.
- Eat organic when possible. Refer to the "dirty dozen" and the "clean ten" lists found at 7SystemsPlan.com.
- Wash your produce. By rinsing your fruit and vegetables in water for 30 seconds, you can remove up to half of the harmful toxins.
- Use natural cleaning products or make your own.
- Switch over to organic toiletries, including shampoo, toothpaste, deodorants, and cosmetics.

To defend your body against the toxins you can't avoid, you'll need to involve all five of your Detox System workers. We'll focus on these one at a time.

Why Your Liver Is Working Against You

Your liver is the team captain of the Detox System. You can remove your spleen, appendix, and tonsils and still live. However, if your liver stops working and you don't get a transplant, you will not live for more than a few days.

This organ is about the size of a football. It's located under your ribs on the right side of your body and is surrounded by a tough capsule.

Liver cells contain enzymes that convert toxins into a form that your body can eliminate. Many toxins tend to behave like fats—they don't dissolve in water. To get rid of these toxins, your body must convert them into water-soluble substances that can be excreted from your body. Every drug, chemical, pesticide, and hormone is broken down by the liver's enzyme pathway.

This process is quite complicated, and it can fail if your liver is not healthy or if your diet is low in certain key nutrients.

The Two Phases of Liver Detox

Imagine that the trash is about to be picked up from your house. You first gather the trash from around the house (Phase I liver detox). Then you put it into bags and take it out (Phase II liver detox). Now your house is clean—the bad stuff is out on the curb.

But what happens if the trash bags never leave the house? You will have a rotten mess that makes everyone in the house miserable and sick. That is what happens when Phase I and Phase II liver detox do not work correctly.

Phase I
The liver combines enzymes (CYP450) with fat-soluble toxins to make them into a compound that can move on to the next phase for elimination from the body. This molecule is now called a reactive intermediary molecule.

At this point, some toxins are harmless, but others can

damage your liver and body. It is imperative that the detox process continues so that the toxins can be eliminated.

Some of the nutrients necessary for this phase include B vitamins, calcium, magnesium, iron, vitamins E and D3, NAC, and indoles from cruciferous vegetables (cabbage, broccoli, cauliflower, and brussels sprouts).

Phase II

Now the liver adds other enzymes (conjugases) to the reactive intermediary molecule to neutralize it and make it water-soluble. The toxin can now be eliminated through the kidneys or moved with the bile into the intestinal tract for elimination.

Some nutrients necessary for this phase include amino acids, calcium, NAC, and MSM. Eggs, cruciferous vegetables, and onions are good sources of sulfur compounds that enhance Phase II.

If your diet is low in any of these key nutrients, Phase I and Phase II detox will not work efficiently and toxins will remain in your body. Consuming adequate amounts of macronutrients and micronutrients as prescribed in the 7 Systems Plan supports optimal liver function.

Be aware that alcohol and some medications (pain medication, statins, acid-blockers, antibiotics, and psychiatric drugs) can injure your liver and impair your detox ability.

Fatty Liver Disease

If your liver has too much fat in it, it will not function correctly. This problem is called fatty liver disease, and it's directly related to obesity. Today, about 30 million Americans have fatty liver disease, and there may be up to 50 million more undiagnosed cases.

There is a close association between obesity, insulin resistance, and fatty liver disease. Where you find one of these problems, you almost invariably find the others:

- Obese individuals have 5 to 15 times the rate of fatty liver disease compared to the non-obese. One study showed that fatty liver disease is present in 57–91% of obese patients![12]
- Up to 85% of type 2 diabetics have fatty livers.[13]
- Even without diabetes, those with an insulin resistance have higher levels of liver fat.

You can develop this disease by having just 20 pounds of fat in the wrong area. People who are apple-shaped (have most of their fat around their belly) have the highest risk. As your abdomen fills up with fat, so does your liver. The capsule that surrounds your liver can stretch, causing some pain or discomfort on your right side under your ribs. If you can feel the enlargement of your liver under your right ribs, that is a warning sign.

Risk factors for fatty liver disease include abdominal obesity, high blood pressure, high cholesterol, low vitamin D, and diabetes. Symptoms of fatty liver disease can include fatigue, weight loss, and nausea. These symptoms typically don't show until the later stages of liver disease.

Fat in your liver impairs its ability to detox adequately. If left untreated, it can lead to cirrhosis and irreversible damage to the liver. It is projected that this will be the number one reason for liver transplants in America in the next 20 years.[14]

Losing belly fat is the most important step to eliminating fatty liver disease. This alone will frequently resolve the problem and allow your liver to repair itself. The 7 Systems Plan has helped many patients restore optimal liver function.

In a recent study, patients with advanced cases of fatty liver disease were placed on a diet and exercise program for one year. The results were remarkable. 90% of those who lost 10% or more of their body weight resolved their condition. Additionally, 45% experienced regression of their liver damage and scarring.[15]

Make sure you're not deficient in vitamin D. It's a significant factor in the progression of fatty liver disease. Keep your blood levels of vitamin D above 50 ng/ml.

How to Get Your Liver Working for You

Though liver damage can be frightening, the steps to heal it are quite simple.

Step 1: Get Tested.

If you think that your liver may be impaired, undergo some lab tests to see how it is functioning. Alkaline phosphatase, alanine aminotransferase (ALT), and aspartate aminotransferase (AST) are measured to screen for liver disease.

Step 2: Eat Right.

Support your liver with cruciferous vegetables. These vegetables are unique because they are rich in sulfur-containing compounds called glucosinolates that support detox and reduce the risk of breast, colon, and lung cancer.[16]

Here is a list to get you started:

- Arugula
- Bok choy
- Broccoli
- Brussels sprouts
- Cabbage
- Cauliflower
- Collard greens
- Kale
- Mustard greens
- Radishes
- Turnips
- Watercress

To find recipes using cruciferous vegetables, visit 7SystemsPlan.com.

Step 3: Take Supplements.

Get your vitamin D3 level in the ideal range and take supplements to support Phase I and Phase II liver detox.

Why Your Kidneys Are Working Against You

In the kidneys, neutralized toxins are filtered out and excreted from your body in urine. This is sometimes referred to as Phase III detox.

This phase does not work well if your body is too acidic. If you have ever taken chemistry, you will recall that some things are acidic (have a low pH) and some things are alkaline (have a high pH). Overeating protein and grains can make your body acidic. This is often the case for overweight people.

Your blood pH should be slightly alkaline—ranging from 7.35 to 7.45. As long as it remains in this range, your chemical, enzymatic, digestive, metabolic, cognitive, immune, and repair processes can work at peak efficiency. Maintaining a healthy blood pH level is critical. If this varies even slightly, you could experience severe health consequences and even death.

To keep your pH from dropping below the critical level, your body holds a reserve of alkaline minerals in your bones. As your pH drops, alkalizing minerals (like calcium) are drawn out of the bones and enter the blood to raise the pH. Over many decades, depletion of the bones' mineral reserves leads to osteopenia or osteoporosis.

If you do not eat healthy foods, this pH regulation process does not function as it should. It is inhibited further by stress, pollutants, very strenuous exercise, illnesses, injuries, drinking water without minerals, a lack of vegetables, and the standard American diet.

At 7SystemsPlan.com, I identify some foods that may be making your body overly acidic. I also list foods that will raise your pH level.

It is important to avoid medications that can damage your kidneys, especially cholesterol medication, pain medications (NSAIDs), antibiotics, diabetic medications, and antacid medications.[17] Considering the amount of these drugs that Americans consume, it's no wonder that so many of us end up on dialysis. Fix your Systems so that you don't need medications.

The Importance of Water

Your kidneys maintain the appropriate balance of water in your body. Babies are 75% water and adults are 60% water. The heart and brain have the most water at 73%. Water is essential for digestion, the absorption of nutrients, and toxin removal. It also aids in circulation, helps control your body temperature, and even lubricates your joints.

You cannot survive for more than a few days without water, but you can survive for many years with insufficient water intake—though it will compromise your overall health.

People tend to dehydrate as they get older, some more than others. Think of it this way:

Aging Drying Dying

People start out like grapes and end up like raisins. Studies show that 75% of Americans are chronically dehydrated. Many vague symptoms and serious medical problems are connected to dehydration.[18]

So, how much water do you need?

Experts vary on the exact amount. Some say half of your weight in ounces per day. Some say eight glasses of water per day. Some say only drink if you are thirsty.

I believe that most people do not drink enough water. As you get older, your thirst signal does not work as well as it should. It is important for people over 50 not to rely on this signal alone for water consumption.

It would be better to err on the high water intake side, especially when you are losing weight. Remember that when fat cells release their fat, the toxins that accumulate in the fat cells are also released. Extra water can flush these toxins from your body.

Many factors determine the amount of water you need:

- What you eat
- How much you sweat
- The temperature
- Caffeine consumption
- Your height and weight

The general rule of thumb is that you need six to eight glasses of good water per day. Some people need even more than this. *When* you drink water is also important. Your body may only be able to use four ounces every 30 minutes. If you drink more than that, it may just pass through your body. Try to drink some water at least every hour.

Here is how to know if you are dehydrated:[19]

- If you pull up the skin on the back of your hand and it stays up like a tent, it is a sign that you are dehydrated.
- If you are urinating less than four to seven times per day, you may be dehydrated.
- If your urine is dark yellow or orange, it is most likely too concentrated; you are not taking in enough fluids. The ideal color for urine is a light yellow. If you are taking B vitamins, it will make your urine turn a brighter yellow.
- If your urine has a strong smell, it could be due to the amount of ammonia in it. Some foods (like asparagus) and even medications can change the look and odor of your urine, so a one-time change should not cause alarm.

Not all water is created equal. Drinking water in many areas of the United States is unsafe. More than 16 million Americans have polyfluoroalkyl PFASs (nonstick chemicals), lead, and per-chlorate (a chemical in explosives) in their water. Because water treatment does not filter out drugs, 10% to 80% of people have painkillers, hormones, antidepressants, antibiotics, cholesterol drugs, and more in their water.[20]

I discourage my patients from drinking tap water or bottled water. If you must drink tap water, leave it out in a glass pitcher for eight hours to release the chlorine. The best thing to do is get a water filtration system.

I suggest that you use a good carbon filter for all your water needs (reverse osmosis and distilled water remove minerals, so they are not my favorites). I have gone through several filters and now only recommend one water filtration system. It has a carbon filter that reduces MTBE, chlorination by-products, PCBs, chloramine, VOCs, heavy metals, and numerous other contaminants. It consistently meets the highest standards. I believe it is the best filter for your needs. It is simple to install, inexpensive, and the best value for your money. See 7SystemsPlan.com for more information.

Water and Weight Loss
In a study published in the *Journal of Obesity*, researchers had people drink 16 ounces of water 30 minutes before their meals. As a result of the experiment, the subjects lost 9 pounds in 12 weeks![21]

Drinking that amount of water before eating takes up space in your stomach and sets off your volume sensor so that you feel full, eat less, and feel more satisfied.

How to Get Your Kidneys Working for You

Step 1: Determine your pH level.

Buy some litmus paper at your local pharmacy or health food store. Use it to check your salivary pH. It should test between 6.8 and 7. If it is below 6.6, you need to work on raising your pH. Your urine pH should fall between 6.5 and 7.25.

You will never fix your pH unless you fix your diet. Follow the 7 Systems Plan. For additional tips to fix your pH, visit 7SystemsPlan.com.

Step 2: Hydrate your body.

- Determine the number of ounces you need in a day. Drink half your body weight in ounces during the weight-loss phase. For the maintenance phase, get at least 60 to 80 ounces a day.
- Purchase a good water filtration system.
- Fill a glass or stainless steel pitcher with water and keep it cold in your refrigerator, ready for drinking.
- Add lemon slices or cucumber to your water to give it some flavor and a fresh scent.
- Buy a glass or stainless steel water bottle with the ounces written on the side to keep track of how much you are drinking.
- Drink 16 ounces of water 30 minutes before meals and experience the benefits of feeling full faster.

Step 3: Regain control of over-the-counter pain medications.

For many people, popping pain pills has become a bad habit. It's something we instinctively reach for whenever we feel pain.

Limiting over-the-counter medications will benefit your kidneys. Gradually lower your dosage and find other ways to deal with headaches and body pains. For long-lasting, drug-free relief, see a chiropractor.

Why Your Colon Is Working Against You

Waste material enters the colon in a mostly liquid form. Bacteria in the colon break down the remaining solids and water is reabsorbed into the bloodstream. The waste then passes on to the rectum where it is stored until removed. Waste is not meant to remain in the colon very long.

Constipation

Of all the problems that happen in the GI tract, constipation is the most common. Many people—physicians included—think that constipation is not a serious problem. They say that if you have a bowel movement every two or three days, you are fine. The truth is that your bowels should move every day or even two or three times per day.

Constipation makes you feel miserable, but that is just the beginning of your troubles. If waste material is left in your colon, it can be reabsorbed by your body, creating a toxic environment. Constipation is known to increase your risk for serious diseases including colon cancer, diverticulosis, and appendicitis. Straining to have a bowel movement can lead to hemorrhoids or tearing of the anus.

If constipation is left unchecked, the result is fecal impaction. Your bowel material can become like concrete and may have to be removed. The number of people who go to the emergency room for constipation has increased dramatically over the last 10 years.

Constipation has many causes. One of the most common is ignoring the urge to have a bowel movement. In your GI tract, you have something called the gastrocolic reflex. Every time you eat, your colon is stimulated to move material out the other end. For some people, this is an immediate reflex, and for others, it can take an hour or two.

Don't ignore this urge when it comes. Sometimes you are too busy or away from home, and you fight the urge. The problem with this is that the urge does not last long, and it may disappear forever if you ignore it long enough.

Other causes of constipation include hypothyroidism, bad bacteria in your gut, laxative abuse, irritable bowel syndrome, antacids, antidepressants, blood pressure medication, and iron supplements.

Another frequent cause of constipation is dehydration. It is imperative that you drink enough water each day to keep the Digestive System working correctly. Water keeps the material in the gut fluid so that it moves through easily. Dry material is harder to move.

Don't forget the fiber. Fiber has no calories or nutrients, and it cannot be digested. However, it is essential. The healthiest fibers come from fruits, vegetables, beans, nuts, and seeds. Processed food has very little, if any, fiber.

You might wonder, "Since there are no nutrients and no calories, why bother to make fiber a part of my diet?"

- Fiber absorbs substantial amounts of water, making it easier for material to move through the bowel. This decreases constipation and straining. People with irritable bowel syndrome relieve their symptoms by consuming more fiber.
- Fiber is an excellent weight-loss tool. It has a bloating effect on your stomach and intestinal tract that helps you feel satisfied with fewer calories. Fiber also binds and absorbs some of the fat in food, preventing it from entering your bloodstream.
- Fiber aids in detox by binding with toxins and excess hormones that your body wants to get rid of. When your liver excretes cholesterol into the intestines, it binds with fiber and is eliminated. This raises HDL (good cholesterol) and lowers LDL (bad cholesterol). If you are not eating enough fiber, cholesterol can be reabsorbed in your intestines and reenter your bloodstream.
- People with high-fiber diets control their blood sugar better than those with low-fiber diets. Fiber has been shown to help both type 1 and type 2 diabetics.
- The prevalence of colon cancer increases in populations that consume less fiber. Fiber has also been shown to lower the risk of pancreatic, endometrial, and many other types of cancer.

- Feeding the beneficial bacteria in your intestinal tract is one of fiber's most important roles. As you eat more fiber, beneficial bacteria increase, and harmful bacteria decrease.

Lots of Fiber:	Lack of Fiber:
Fiber feeds good gut bacteria	No food for the good gut bacteria
Short-chain fatty acids produced (heals gut)	No short-chain fatty acids produced (no healing)
Hormones released	No hormones released
Appetite turned off = Weight loss	Appetite turned on = weight gain

The people who live the longest consume between 40 or more grams of fiber per day. Americans consume approximately 15 grams per day.[22] I recommend that my patients get at least 35 grams. Don't increase your grain intake to get fiber. If you are eating lots of fruits, vegetables, and beans, you should be able to hit at least 35 grams.

How to Get Your Colon Working for You

Here are three steps to eliminate the causes of constipation.

Step 1: Increase your fiber intake.

Aim for at least 35 grams per day. 100 grams would be better. Eat fruits, vegetables, legumes, nuts, and seeds on a daily basis. If you are having trouble consuming enough fiber, get the PGX fiber supplement from your local health food store. Take 2–5 grams with a big glass of water before each meal.

Step 2: Limit certain foods.

Red meat, dairy, chips, frozen dinners, cookies, bananas (unripe), and fried foods cause constipation.

Step 3: Take supplements.

Magnesium citrate, omega-3, probiotics, and vitamin C improve colon function.

Visit 7SystemsPlan.com for additional tools.

Why Your Lungs Are Working Against You

Every time you breathe, you inhale and exhale poison gases. Each year, 6.5 million people worldwide die prematurely from indoor and outdoor air pollution.[23] Since most Americans spend up to 90% of their time indoors, you should be most concerned about indoor air pollution. It may be 2 to 5 times—and up to 100 times—higher than outdoor pollution, according to the EPA.[24]

To be healthy, you must breathe clean air, but it's also important to breathe correctly. Most people are taught to breathe deeply from the belly. While there is a time and place for that, if you breathe too deeply, it can lead to something called hyperventilation syndrome.

It is very important that you use your nose when you breathe and not your mouth. Breathing through your mouth can bring in too much oxygen and make your blood carbon dioxide level drop dangerously low. Carbon dioxide has many important functions in your bloodstream. Less carbon dioxide in your blood makes your pH more alkaline. As you have learned, it is critical for your blood pH to remain within a very narrow window.

Excess oxygen causes a constriction of your blood vessels, resulting in decreased blood flow to the heart, brain, and muscles. This can lead to irregular heartbeats, dizziness, and lightheadedness.

Your in-breath should be shorter than your out-breath. This will help you relax and maintain healthy levels of oxygen and carbon dioxide in your blood. Many people breathe up to three times more than they should, contributing to all sorts of health problems. Even during exercise, it is important that you breathe through your nose with your mouth closed as much as possible.

Over breathing, or "the disease of deep breathing," can be a habit that is difficult to break. How do you know if you are over breathing?

If you breathe through your mouth, sigh frequently, take large breaths before talking, sniff or yawn often, or have sleep apnea, you may have this problem. Over breathing can cause heart, neurological, respiratory, muscular, gastrointestinal, and psychological problems.

The nose is the most underused organ in your body. It performs approximately 30 different jobs: It humidifies the air you breathe in, checks for harmful odors, and sends signals directly to your brain.

Breathing softly and calmly is important. One of the nose's most vital jobs is to normalize your breathing rate. You should normally take in about 10 to 12 breaths per minute. Patrick McKeown, a well-known authority on the subject, says, "Breathe light to breathe right." If you breathe through your mouth instead of your nose, you're putting your health at risk.

Refer to 7SystemsPlan.com for a summary of Patrick McKeown's Buteyko breathing method.[25]

How to Get Your Lungs Working for You

Step 1: Exercise your lungs each day.

Exercise is a proven way to increase your lung function and capacity.

Step 2: Shut your mouth.

Practice breathing correctly using your nose.

Step 3: Eliminate airborne toxins in your environment.

Avoid these toxins:

- Tobacco smoke
- Volatile organic compounds from paints

- Aerosol sprays and household cleaners
- Pesticides
- Phthalates from vinyl flooring and personal care products
- Pollutants from pressure-treated wood products
- Radon gas
- Mold

Add these elements to your daily breathing:

- An air purification system
- Houseplants that remove indoor toxins[26]

Why Your Skin Is Working Against You

Your skin is the largest organ in your body at an estimated 22 square feet of skin per person. Your skin contains millions of sweat glands that help regulate body temperature and eliminate toxins.

Skin is a valuable part of your Detox System, but it only works if you sweat. In one study, blood, urine, and sweat were collected from 20 individuals and analyzed for approximately 120 various compounds, including toxins. The findings were revealing. Sweating appears to be a good method for eliminating many toxic elements from the human body, and some toxins are best excreted through sweating.[27]

Your skin doesn't only excrete toxins—it absorbs them. This is why it's so important to be aware of what your skin touches. One drop of mercury on your skin can be fatal. Toxins from cosmetics, perfumes, antiperspirants, cleaning supplies, chlorine, and many other common substances can enter your body through your skin.

How to Get Your Skin Working for You

Step 1: Get sweaty frequently.

I suggest getting sweaty with exercise because of its other health benefits, but saunas can also be helpful.

Step 2: Do not use antibacterial soaps.

Use regular soap and apply only to the parts of your body where it is needed. You do not want to remove beneficial bacteria.

Step 3: Limit the things that come into contact with your skin.

Use natural cosmetics, deodorant, and cleaning supplies.

Quick Recap:

- Assume you are toxic, because everyone is.
- Being toxic will make you gain weight, not feel well, and develop diseases.
- Following The 7 System Plan will help you detox.
- You must limit your toxic exposure if you want to be healthy.
- You need to support the five main workers in your Detox System.

Proven Steps to Fix Your Detox System:

(Check these off as you complete them. Join our free 7 Systems Plan Community for additional support and encouragement: 7SystemsPlan.com.)

☐ Limit toxin exposure from all sources.

☐ Drink enough good water.

☐ Identify the weak link in your Detox System and support it.

☐ Try the 10-day detox program at 7SystemsPlan.com.

Supplements to Support Your Detox System

If you suspect you have toxin problems, you may want to consider integrating a few proven products to support your Detox System.

Dynamic Detox is a product that Beth used for metabolic detox, alkalization (increased pH), and heavy metal elimination. It supports detox Phases I, II, and III.

If you want to try the 10-day detox program that started Beth's health journey, you can find it at 7SystemsPlan.com and see Appendix A, Part Five, for more information.

Detox System Lab Tests

Simple At-Home Test: Eye, Joint, and Stool Test

Check under your eyes for puffy dark circles, check your joints for multiple pain areas, and check your stool for a foul smell. All of these may indicate a malfunctioning Detox System.

Liver

- Elevated liver enzymes (Alkaline phosphatase, ALT, and AST) may indicate fatty liver disease or impaired liver function.
- GGT greater than 40 IU/L may indicate toxicity or disease of the liver or bile duct.

Kidney

- Decreased GFR, increased creatinine, or protein in the urine may indicate that your kidneys are not functioning optimally.

Colon

- Less than daily bowel movements may show that you have a sluggish colon that could be absorbing toxins.

Lung

- Decreased lung function will impair your ability to eliminate toxins as you breath. Spirometry is the most common lung function test. It measures how much and how quickly you can move air out of your lungs.

Skin

- Lack of perspiration means that you aren't eliminating toxins through your sweat.

Other Tests

These test results may also indicate toxicity:

- HDL lower than 30 mg/dL
- BMI greater than 27
- Vitamin D less than 30 ng/mL

Visit 7SystemsPlan.com for more of my lab test recommendations.

Conclusion

Congratulations. You've made it all the way to the conclusion, which is no small feat. If your body could speak, it would thank you.

Let me remind you how far you've come. In the Introduction, you discovered how the 7 Systems Plan offers a new way of life that comes from a new way of thinking: Weight-loss problems and disease exist when one or more of your Systems are not functioning correctly.

In this book, our strategy has been three-fold: We evaluated your Systems, identified imbalances and malfunctions, and then optimized your Systems.

The 7 System Strategy

Evaluate → Identify → Optimize

By now, you're aware that your body is a well-designed creation. Every System in it—if running properly—has a job to do.

However, if a System is compromised, your entire body could grind to a halt.

Debbie agrees.

You might remember her from Chapter Two. She's the lady who wanted to lose weight and get healthy. She came in for testing and recommendations but did not have the knowledge provided in this book. She didn't have the support or accountability to succeed either. She abandoned her program, and her diabetes worsened—eventually putting her in a diabetic coma. She spent weeks in the hospital.

It always bothers me when I have a patient fail to regain his or her health. As I was writing this book, I called Debbie and asked her if she would read *7 Systems Plan* as I was writing it. I wanted her feedback on each chapter. I also asked her to join my 7 Systems Plan Online Course since she lives four hours from my office.

Debbie agreed, and her amazing transformation surprised us both.

In Chapter One, she learned the importance of silencing the angry fat in her Structural System that was sabotaging her health. She restarted the 7 Systems Plan and implemented FMDs to speed up her progress and get her body under control.

In Chapter Two, she realized that her Digestive System was the source of many of her health problems. She integrated the recommended functional food and probiotics for weight loss. She also added helpers to her will power to insure her success.

In Chapter Three, she discovered the importance of moving key macronutrients and micronutrients through her Delivery System. She eliminated the bad carbohydrates that were sabotaging her health, added quality nutrients to her diet, and began to enjoy eating vegetables.

In Chapter Four, she recognized that her mitochondria had been compromised, decreasing her body's ability to produce energy. With the new food she was eating, a new exercise program, and no more late-night eating, she ramped up her Energy System.

In Chapter Five, she saw how her Communication System was sabotaging her efforts, and she took steps to correct her hormone problems. She also identified food addiction issues, which she eliminated.

In Chapter Six, she came to grips with her body's chronic inflamed state. She added more good fats to her diet to support her Defense System, and she eliminated the things that were hindering it.

In Chapter Seven, she understood the finer points of her Detox System and how she could leverage it to work for her instead of against her.

The online course also gave Debbie the support and encouragement she needed to experience health. The results were amazing:

1. In just six weeks, she lost 20 pounds. She continued the 7 Systems Plan and is now down by 60 pounds.
2. She reinoculated her gut with good bacteria that will help keep her healthy.
3. She started enjoying real food.
4. Her energy increased tremendously, allowing her to enjoy life again.
5. Within days of starting the 7 Systems Plan, she was able to reduce her insulin injections from 50 units a day to 0. She is now off her long list of medications for high cholesterol and kidney failure, PPIs for acid reflux, insulin for diabetes, and more.
6. She "put out the fire," calming down the inflammation in her body.
7. Her Detox System was finally able to do its job.

She is now healthy, happy, and enjoying her life again.

Your future results can be just as profound.

This book was designed to help you evaluate, identify, and optimize your compromised Systems. Once you get them working for you instead of against you, you'll have amazing health transformations, lose weight, and heal chronic illness.

Now that you've completed the book, I want to invite you to take the next step and start making this a lifestyle. The 7 Systems Plan Online Course and Community will help you make fast progress toward weight loss, health, and vitality.

Isn't it time to get your life back?

Appendix Order

Appendix A: Resources

Part One
Tips to make the 7 Systems Plan work for you
What to Eat and How Much to Eat
Choosing Your Fish

Part Two
Determine Your Daily Caloric Need
Choose the Number of Calories You Will Eat per Day

Part Three
Using Your Food Journal

Part Four
Develop Your Success Plan

Part Five
Functional Foods
Vitamins for Every Adult

Part Six
Restricted Calorie Menus
300-Calorie Meals in About 5 Minutes
Fast-Mimicking Diet Menus

- 17-Hour Fast
- 23-Hour Fast
- 5:2 Plan

Part Seven
Simple At-Home Fitness Test
Aerobic Exercise Zone
Whole-Body Weight Lifting Interval Routine

Appendix B: The 7 Systems Online Course

Appendix A: Resources

Here is a quick overview of what to do with this appendix:

1. Read the tips to make the 7 Systems Plan work for you.
2. Use the shopping list to stock up on real food.
3. Determine your daily caloric need.
4. Choose number of calories you will eat per day and determine the servings that you are allowed from each food
   group.
5. Use your food journal.
6. Begin by eating three meals per day.
7. Start your exercise program.

Part One

Tips to Make the 7 Systems Plan Work for You:

- **Finish reading the entire book** if you have not done so already. The more knowledgeable you are, the better health choices you will make and the more successful you will be in achieving your goals.
- **Use the shopping list** to load up your cupboards and refrigerator with real food.
- Find a way to eat vegetables in every meal. Go crazy with salads. Visit 7SystemsPlan.com for tips on easy, enjoyable ways to eat more vegetables.
- **Plan your eating for the next day or the whole week if you can.** If you're like many people, you get home after a long day and have to figure out what's for dinner. I know it is very easy to make poor food choices when this happens. Prepare meals ahead of time and have them in your refrigerator or freezer ready to go. I have patients who make healthy pizzas with cauliflower rice for the crusts and freeze them for future use.
- **Mix it up.** After a few weeks of eating the same food, you may become bored and get off your success plan. Try something new every week. I encourage my patients to try one new recipe each week. If you find one that you like, put it on a list of meals that you make every two weeks.
- **Keep it simple.** If you have to spend two hours each day on food prep, you are doomed to fail. My suggestions and recipes are simple and fast. If one of them does take longer to make, prepare enough for three meals.
- **Focus on the actions** that you are taking each day to accomplish your health goals. After you get through the first 7–10 days, focus on how much better you feel, how much more energy you have, and how much better your brain is working.
- **If you need to lose weight, watch the scale.** If weighing every day will discourage you when your weight does not go down, then weigh once a week. You must understand that your weight will fluctuate up and down even if you are doing the right things. If this will not bother you, weigh daily. If the scale

reading doesn't change after a week, that is not a problem. No change after two weeks means that you are not following the 7 Systems Plan accurately or you need to adjust your methods.

- **Use the success plan sheet** to set up your team of helpers.
- **Set one-week goals,** monthly goals, and final goals.
- **If you fail one day, get back to it.** Almost all of my patients have setbacks at times. The ones who are successful are those who learn from their mistakes and keep at it. Think progress— not perfection.
- **Continue reading through Appendix A,** and I will walk you through exactly what to do.
- **Visit 7SystemsPlan.com** for more help and resources.

What to Eat and How Much to Eat:
Shopping List with Food Groups and Serving Sizes

To be successful on this plan, you must keep your house loaded with the right foods. Take this list and go shopping! (See 7SystemsPlan.com for a printable version.) Circle the foods you are going to buy. You can also use this list to check the serving size and calories of each food item.

Legumes

Serving size: 1/2 cup cooked, or as indicated (1 serving = approximately 110 calories)

- **Beans**: black, butter, cannellini, garbanzo, great northern, pinto, kidney, lima, navy, mung, fat-free refried, green soy
- **Lentils**: beluga, French, and red
- **Bean soups**, 3/4 cup
- **Hummus**, 1/4 cup
- **Peas**: split green or yellow peas

Vegetables—Low-GI

Serving size: 1/2 cup. Servings unlimited. Fresh juices made from these are allowed. (1 serving = approximately 10–25 calories)

- **Cruciferous**: broccoli, brussels sprouts, cabbages (all types), cauliflower, radishes
- **Greens**: beet greens, bok choy, collard greens, escarole, kale, mustard greens, Swiss chard, watercress
- **Lettuce/Mixed greens**: arugula, endive, radicchio, red and green leaf, romaine, spinach
- **Mushrooms**
- **Other vegetables:** artichokes, asparagus, celery, chives, cucumbers, dill pickles, eggplants, garlic, green beans, kelp,

leeks, mixed vegetable juices, okra, onions, peppers, radishes, snow peas, tomatoes, water chestnuts (5 whole)
- **Salsa** (sugar-free)
- **Sprouts**: alfalfa, broccoli or radish sprouts, bamboo shoots, etc.
- **Squash**: spaghetti, summer, yellow, zucchini

Vegetables—Medium-GI

Serving size: 1/2 cup, or as indicated (1 serving = approximately 45 calories)

- **Beets**, 1 cup
- **Carrots**, 1/2 cup cooked, 2 medium raw, or 12 baby carrots
- **Pumpkins**, 2/3 cup
- **Rutabagas,** 1 cup
- **Sweet potatoes or yams**, 1/2 medium
- **Turnips**, 1 1/2 cup
- **Winter squash**: acorn, butternut
- **Yukon Gold potato**, 1/2 medium

Concentrated Proteins

Serving size: 3–4 oz. cooked, or as indicated. Meat, poultry, and fish should be broiled, baked, or roasted. Keep cheese intake low due to saturated fat. (1 serving = approximately 150 calories)

Best

- **More low-GI vegetables** (1 frozen package of spinach has 10g of protein)
- **Tofu**, 8 oz. or 1 cup (fresh), or 3.5 oz. cube
- **Tempeh**, 3 oz. or 1/2 cup
- **Soy or veggie burger**, 4 oz.
- **Fish** (wild-caught only): salmon, sardines, mackerel (not king), shellfish (3 oz. fresh or 3/4 cup canned in water; if canned in oil, drain well)

- **Beef, lamb, or chicken** (free-range only)
- **Functional Foods** (available at 7SystemsPlan.com)

Good

- **Beef** (very lean)
- **Other fish** (wild-caught and low in mercury)
- **Eggs** (cage-free, organic), 2 whole
- **Egg substitute**, 2/3 cup
- **Poultry**: chicken or Cornish hen (breast only), turkey
- **Leg of lamb** (lean roast)
- **Cottage cheese** (nonfat or low-fat), 3/4 cup
- **Ricotta** (part skim or nonfat), 1/2 cup
- **Mozzarella** (part skim or nonfat), 2 oz. or 1/2 cup shredded
- **Parmesan**, 4 tablespoon grated

Nuts and Seeds

Serving size as indicated (1 serving = approximately 100 calories)

- **Almonds, Brazil nuts, cashews, hazelnuts, macadamia nuts**, 10–12 whole nuts
- **Walnut or Pecan**, 7–8 halves
- **Pistachios, sunflower seeds, pumpkin seeds, sesame seeds**, 2 tablespoon
- **Nut butter**, 1 tablespoon made from the above nuts
- **Peanut butter** (this is my least favorite), 1 tablespoon refrigerated and no sugar added

Fats

Serving size: 1 teaspoon, or as indicated (1 serving = approximately 40 calories). Always use avocados and olives as your first pick.

- **Avocado**, 1/8

- **Olives,** 8–10 medium
- **Walnut oil or avocado oil**
- **Extra virgin coconut oil** (use for high heat stove top cooking)
- **Cold-pressed extra virgin olive oil** (for cooking and dressing)
- **Mayonnaise** (made with avocado oil), 2 teaspoons

Fruit

Serving size as indicated (1 serving = approximately 80 calories)

Berries

- **Blackberries or blueberries,** 1 cup
- **Raspberries or strawberries,** 1 1/2 cups

Other fruits

- **Apples,** 1 medium
- **Apricots,** 3 medium, 1/4 cup dried
- **Cantaloupe,** 1/2 medium
- **Cherries,** 15
- **Clementines,** 2
- **Fresh figs,** 2
- **Grapes,** 15
- **Honeydew melon,** 1/4 small
- **Kiwifruits,** 2 medium
- **Mango,** 1/2 medium
- **Nectarines,** 2 small
- **Oranges,** 1 large
- **Peaches,** 2 small
- **Pears,** 1 medium
- **Plums,** 2 small
- **Tangerines,** 2 small
- **Watermelon,** 2 cups

Dairy

If you can, skip this group and add more to the fat group. Serving size: 6 oz., or as indicated (1 serving = approximately 80 calories)

- **Butter or ghee** (pasture-raised, organic), 2 1/2 teaspoon
- **Buttermilk**
- **Yogurt** (plain, homemade is best), 4 oz.
- **Almond, hemp, coconut milk, soy** (unsweetened)

Grain

Serving size: 1/2 cup cooked, or as indicated (1 serving = approximately 75–100 calories)

- **Amaranth, teff, or quinoa**
- **Rice**: basmati or other brown rice, wild
- **Barley, buckwheat groats, or millet**
- **Bulgur** (cracked wheat)
- **Popcorn**, 2 cups popped
- **Whole oats**, 1/3 cup raw, 3/4 cup cooked
- **Whole wheat, spelt, or kamut berries**
- **100% whole wheat, spelt, or kamut pasta**
- **Crackers** (small whole-grain crackers), 8
- **Breads**: 1 slice mixed whole grain or 100% whole rye, 1/2 whole-wheat tortilla or pita, 2 small or 1 large low-carb tortilla

Beverages

8 glasses per day

- **Water** (filtered)
- **Coffee** (2 cups per day limit)
- **Herbal or green teas**
- **Sparkling or mineral water**

Choosing Your Fish

Remember to choose fish that are high in omega-3 and low in mercury.

Omega-3 Content in Fish:

Type of fish	Total omega-3 content per 3.5 ounces (100 grams)
Mackerel	2.6 (Canadian & Atlantic only)
Trout, lake	2.0
Herring	1.7
Salmon	1.5
Sardines, canned	1.5
Sturgeon, Atlantic	1.5
Whitefish, lake	1.5
Anchovies	1.4
Bluefish	1.2
Bass, striped	0.8
Trout	0.6
Halibut, Pacific	0.5
Pollock	0.5
Sturgeon	0.4
Bass, freshwater	0.3
Catfish	0.3
Ocean perch	0.3
Flounder	0.2
Haddock	0.2
Snapper, red	0.2
Sole	0.1

Mercury in Fish

High Mercury

- Bluefish
- Grouper
- Mackerel (Spanish, Gulf)
- Sea Bass (Chilean)
- Tuna (canned albacore)
- Tuna (yellowfin)

Highest Mercury

Avoid eating these:

- Mackerel (king)
- Marlin
- Orange roughy
- Shark
- Swordfish
- Tilefish
- Tuna (bigeye, ahi)

Part Two

Determine Your Daily Caloric Need

As a general rule for weight loss, I start female patients on 1,300 calories and men on 1,600–1,800. If you want a more accurate number, use the following formula to figure out how many calories you need per day to maintain the same weight. Subtract 30% if you want to lose weight.

For an accurate estimate of ideal weight:

- Females calculate 100 pounds for the first 5 feet in height, plus 5 pounds for each inch after that. So, if you are 5' 4", your ideal weight would be 100 + 20 = 120 pounds.

  Males calculate 106 pounds for the first 5 feet and add 6 pounds for each additional inch. So, a 5' 10" male would have an ideal weight of 106 + 60 = 166 pounds.

This is your ideal body weight unless you have a larger-than-average skeletal structure. To determine if you have a large frame, place your thumb and first finger around your wrist. If they can touch, you have an average frame. If not, your ideal weight will be higher than this estimate.

- Next, multiply your ideal body weight by 10 to get your BMR (basal metabolic rate, or resting calorie requirement).

  - Keep in mind that if you have a large frame, this is not accurate, and your BMR will be higher.
  - 5' 4" female with average frame = 120 ideal weight × 10 = 1,200 BMR
  - 5' 10" male with average frame = 166 ideal weight × 10 = 1,660 BMR

- Add 30% for the calories you burn up with daily activities
  - If you have a sedentary life, this percentage will be lower.
  - If you have an active life, this percentage will be higher.

- Add calories burned up from exercise

  - Be realistic with this.

- The total of Steps 1 through 4 equals your calories burned per day. Consuming this amount will keep your weight the same, and consuming less will make it go down (though remember, not all calories are equal). So, a 5' 4" female has a 1,200 (BMR) + 360 (30%) + 200 (exercise) = 1,760 (total calories burned per day).
- Subtract 30% from this number (1,760) to find the number of calories to consume per day for weight loss. 30% of 1,760 calories = 528.

  So, 1,760 – 528 = 1,232 calories per day.

Choose the Number of Calories You Will Eat per Day

Once you have chosen, look at the number of servings you are allowed from each group. Use this to fill out your food journal each day.

	1,000 Calorie	1,300 Calorie	1,600 Calorie	1,900 Calorie
Concentrated Protein	1	1-2	2-3	2-3
Legumes	1	1	2	2
Dairy/Dairy Alternative (Optional)	0	0	1	1
Nuts and Seeds	1	1-2	2	3
Vegetables— Low-GI	6+ minimum 6+ ideal	6+ minimum 6+ ideal	6+ minimum 8+ ideal	6+ minimum 8+ ideal
Vegetables— Med-GI	0-1	0-1	1	1-2
Fruits	1-2	1-2	2	2
Grains	0-1	0-1	0-2	0-2
Healthy Fats	3	4	5	6
Functional Food 1 serving = 1 scoop	1	2	2	2

Part Three

Using Your Food Journal

As you go throughout your day, fill out your food journal on paper or in an app. I highly recommend that you use the paper version the first month (to make the process much easier). Go to 7SystemsPlan.com for a printable multiday version.

Here is the daily food journal process:

1. Record the date and the hours of sleep you had the night before.
2. Record everything you eat (be exact) and skip snacks (if you absolutely cannot skip snacks in the beginning, you can make an exception, but wean yourself off of them).
3. Record your total calories for the day.
4. Record the ounces of water you drank (ideally at least 4 oz. every 30 minutes).
5. Circle the type of exercise you did, and record the duration of each exercise.
6. Circle the number of servings from each food group at the bottom of the sheet. Strive to eat the correct number of servings from each group every day. (See "What to Eat and How Much to Eat" in Appendix A, Part One, to know how many you should be eating.) If you are not using a functional food, increase your protein, oil, and legume consumption.
7. Record the stress reduction technique you used today (see Chapter Five).
8. Record how you felt today; be honest.
9. If you did well, put a star at the top of the page.

Food Journal

Date:
Hours of Sleep:

First Meal Time:

Second Meal Time:

Third Meal Time:

Total Calories:

Ounces of water
60, 70, 80, 90, 100, 110, 120

Exercise
Stretch, Weight Lifting, Aerobic, Interval
Minutes:

Low-sugar veg: 1 2 3 4 5 6 7+   Nuts: 1 2 3

Med-sugar veg: 0-2   Legumes: 1 2

Fruit: 1 2   Fats: 1 2 3 4

Protein: 1 2 3   Grain: 0-2

Functional Food: 1 2   Vitamins 1

Stress Technique:

Meal Prep Done for the Next Day: Yes No

How You Felt Today:

Part Four

Develop Your Success Plan

Identify your willpower helpers (refer to Chapter Two for suggestions). Do not skip this step! It will increase your chances of success significantly.

Helper #1: Desire

Here, on a 3x5 card, or on your phone, list what you want to do, and be specific:

   1.
   2.
   3.
   4.

List why you want to do it:

   1.
   2.
   3.
   4.

Helper #2: Skills

List how you are going to acquire new skills and abilities:

   1.
   2.
   3.
   4.

Helper #3: Cheering Section

Identify the people who are going to be your cheering section:

1.
2.
3.
4.

Identify the people who may hinder you:

1.
2.
3.
4.

What will you do to prevent problems with those people?

1.
2.

Helper #4: Coach

Identify the people who will be your coaches or hold you accountable.

1.
2.

Helper #5: Rewards and Incentives

What will your rewards and incentives be for hitting your goals?

1.
2.
3.
4.

What specific events or times can you link your goals to?

1.
2.
3.

Helper #6: Health-Friendly Environment

What do you need to remove from your house and workplace?

1.
2.
3.
4.

What are you going to replace those with?

1.
2.
3.
4.

Part Five

Functional Foods

For the last 15 years, I have used functional foods—as meal replacements or as additions to the diet—to help my patients support their Systems and lose weight.

So, what is a functional food?

A functional food is a dynamic plant-based food that has the macronutrients (fats, carbs, proteins) and micronutrients (vitamins and minerals) necessary to help you achieve your health goals.

Why do I use functional foods?

- They help Systems return to optimal function quicker.
- They speed up weight loss.
- They are convenient, tasty, and easy to use.
- They can be a low-cost, low-calorie meal replacement.
- They help maintain progress.

How do you get functional foods?

These products and vitamins are available from approved health-care providers and at 7SystemsPlan.com.

Which functional food do you need?

If you have a specific System that is causing your weight and health problems, use the appropriate functional food (as a meal replacement or supplement) to support that System.

My favorite functional foods and supplements—and the ones I use the most in my clinic—are Dynamic Daily Meal, Dynamic Cardio-Metabolic, and Dynamic Inflam-Eze. These are available in several tasty flavors.

These functional foods can be used alone; just add 1 scoop to 8 oz. of cold water, shake or blend, and then enjoy. You can also add other food to the shake. Here are two of my favorite recipes:

All Berry Delight

- 8 oz. unsweetened almond milk
- 1 scoop functional food
- 1/4 cup frozen raspberries
- 1/4 cup frozen blackberries
- 1/4 cup frozen strawberries
- 1/4 cup frozen dark cherries
- 1 tablespoon flax or chia seeds
- 4 ice cubes

Blend well in a blender.

Veggie Wonder

This is an easy way to raise your vegetable intake:

- 8 oz. unsweetened almond milk
- 1 scoop functional food
- 1/2 banana
- 2 large handfuls of baby spinach (or frozen spinach)
- 1 handful of kale (stems removed)
- 1 tablespoon flax or chia seeds

Blend well in a blender.

See 7SystemsPlan.com for 30 more tasty options.

Functional Foods for Every System

Here are the functional foods and supplements that I use to help my patients lose weight and fix their Systems. At 7SystemsPlan. com, I have more detailed information and the benefits.

Structural System
Dynamic Daily Meal
The product I use to support the Structural System is Dynamic Daily Meal. This is my favorite functional food. It is a nutritious protein drink to support your Structural System with phytonutrients, vitamins, minerals, and branch chain amino acids (BCAAs), which help with muscle growth.

Dynamic Daily Meal is formulated to nutritionally support a healthy body composition (fat, muscle, and bone).

Digestive System

Dynamic GI Restore
The product I use to support the Digestive System is Dynamic GI Restore. It is a functional food formulated to provide specialized macronutrient and micronutrient support for patients with compromised gut function and digestive disorders, including malabsorption.

Delivery System
A healthy Delivery System requires control of lipids and blood sugar. I use the product below to help patients who have problems with this System.

Dynamic Cardio-Metabolic
This is a functional food formulated to provide specialized nutritional support within a nutritional management program for lipid issues. As part of a heart-healthy eating plan, the addition of plant sterols/stanols has been shown to lead to beneficial changes in LDL cholesterol in individuals with hypercholesterolemia.

This functional food is also formulated for the nutritional management of glucose response. It is designed for individuals who may need additional support in controlling their blood sugar levels.

Energy System
I use two products to support patients' Energy Systems: Dynamic Daily Meal and Cellular Energy

Dynamic Daily Meal
This functional food provides nutritional support for patients with sarcopenia (the age-associated loss of skeletal muscle mass). This advanced formula provides essential amino acids, including added leucine, to support the healthy aging of skeletal muscle and to help address sarcopenia.

Cellular Energy
This product is designed to support the healthy function of your Energy System. It is formulated with efficacious amounts of several energy-supporting ingredients, including coenzyme Q10 (CoQ10), acetyl L-carnitine (ALCAR), N-acetyl L-cysteine (NAC), alpha-lipoic acid (ALA), and grape seed extract.

Communication System
For patients with elevated blood sugar or insulin, I use the Dynamic Cardio-Metabolic described above. For support of estrogen metabolism, I use Dynamic Hormone Balance.

Dynamic Hormone Balance
This is a powdered dietary supplement with a pea and rice protein base that has evidence-based ingredients that support healthy estrogen balance.

Defense System
For problems with inflammation in the gut or other areas, I use Dynamic Inflam-Eze functional food. To support a healthy gastrointestinal tract, I use Dynamic GI Restore. I also suggest a product called PRM Resolve to support immune response. For occasional sleeplessness that can impair the Defense System, try GoodNight.

Dynamic Inflam-Eze
This functional food is formulated to provide strategic macronutrient and micronutrient support for patients with compromised
gut function resulting from inflammatory bowel disease, including ulcerative colitis and Crohn's disease.

Dynamic GI Integrity
This product is designed to provide gastrointestinal nutritional
support. The formula is uniquely designed to aid in promoting
the growth of beneficial bacteria by including prebiotic nutrients
combined with readily digestible macronutrients.

PRM Resolve
This is a revolutionary nutritional product developed through
advanced fractionation technology featuring standardized levels
of pro-resolving mediators found in fish oil. It is designed to
support the body's natural capacity to respond to physical challenges and resolve physical stress.

GoodNight
This sleep and relaxation formula features melatonin, key herbs,
and minerals. This novel formula delivers 5 mg of melatonin per
serving to relieve occasional sleeplessness, complemented by
four concentrated plant extracts to promote a sense of calm and
minerals to target muscle relaxation.

Detox System
The product I use to support the Detox System is Dynamic
Detox.

Dynamic Detox
This functional food is formulated to deliver advanced, specialized nutritional support for Phase I, II, and III detoxification.

10-Day Detox
Dynamic Detox for Metabolic Detoxification Program
My 10-day program featuring Dynamic Detox is designed to enhance the body's natural metabolic detoxification process while providing adequate fuel for both cleansing and other daily activities—providing energy and support for overall well-being. Many people benefit from completing a 10-day metabolic detoxification program two to three times a year.

The 10-day program is ideal for anyone wanting to benefit from an occasional "Spring Cleaning" or somebody who eats a reasonably healthy diet, exercises regularly, and manages stress adequately. It is also ideal for individuals who scored >50 on the Metabolic Detoxification Questionnaire (see 7SystemsPlan. com for the questionnaire).

Vitamins for Every Adult:

Essential Multi
One capsule per day takes you beyond basic wellness support. It has a proprietary blend of highly potent herbal extracts and phytonutrients with scientifically tested biological activity to support cellular health.

Benefits:

- Intelligent blend of highly-concentrated nutrients—to impact cell signaling to communicate healthy messages throughout the body
- Enhanced with select bioactive plant compounds—including lutein, zeaxanthin, lycopene, and resveratrol
- Optimized with essential vitamins and minerals—for multidimensional health support

D3 10,000 with K2
D3 10,000 with K2 provides ultra-concentrated levels of vitamin D3 designed to quickly replenish vitamin D status. This formula also provides active forms of vitamin K2 to complement the activity of vitamin D. Take a minimum of one per week and a maximum of three per week (have a lab test to check your levels; stay at 50 ng/ml).

Benefits:

- Vitamin D promotes healthy bone formation and mineralization and supports immune and cardiovascular health
- Supplies active forms of vitamin K2—designed for greater bioavailability
- Vitamin K is a key vitamin in the metabolism of bone proteins

- Solubilized in oil—to promote better absorption in the digestive tract

Omega Pure EPA-DHA 720 (omega-3)
This supplement offers advanced support for cardiovascular, immune, and joint health. It contains both important omega-3 families (EPA and DHA). Taking a minimum of 2,000 mg. 4,000 mg per day (3–6 pills) is ideal.

UltraBiotic Integrity
This probiotic is designed to help support body weight regulation by delivering targeted probiotic support as Bifidobacterium lactis B-420, which has been shown to help control body fat and body weight. Take this daily (on an empty stomach).

UltraBiotic Daily Multi-Strain
This probiotic provides multidimensional support for both the upper and lower GI tract for digestive and immune health. This concentrated formula supplies a proprietary blend of seven beneficial probiotic strains. Take this daily (on an empty stomach). If you do not have weight problems, this may be the best option.

NutriDyn has had no bearing on the content of this book, and all opinions in the text are those of Dr. Luse. All content from NutriDyn's materials is used with permission.

Part Six

Restricted Calorie Menus

Here are sample menus for getting started on the 7 Systems Plan. Menu one gives you 1,300 calories and menu 2 gives you 1600 calories. See 7SystemsPlan.com for more menus.

Menu 1

Breakfast (230 cal.)
Berry Shake

- 1 scoop functional food—150 cal.
- 1 cup berries—80 cal.

Lunch (680 cal.)
Raw carrots and celery—50 cal.
1/4 cup Hummus dip—110 cal.
Tasty Burger—380 cal.

- 1 veggie or bean burger patty—120 cal.
- 2 teaspoon avocado oil mayo—80 cal.
- 2 slices tomato—6 cal.
- Ketchup (no sugar added)—4 cal.
- 1 slice whole-grain bread—70 cal.

6 sweet potato fries—40 cal.
Functional food—150 cal.

Dinner (510 Cal.)
Roasted chicken and vegetables—370 cal.

- 3 oz. roasted chicken—200 cal.
- 1 cup roasted beets—50 cal.
- 1 cup roasted brussels sprouts—40 cal.
- 2 teaspoon oil—80 cal. (sprinkle over the vegetables and rice and add seasonings)

1 cup cauliflower rice—40 cal.
Walnut or Pecan Halves, 7–8—100 cal.

Total calories for the day: 1,370

Menu 2

Breakfast 330
Berry Delight Shake

- 1 scoop functional food 150 cal.
- 1 1/2 tablespoons chia seeds 100 cal.
- 1 cup berries 80 cal.

Lunch 657
Chicken corn tortilla

- Tortilla 60 cal.
- 4 oz. diced chicken breast 250 cal.
- Black beans ½ cup 110 cal.
- 1/4 cup hummus 100
- Guacamole 1/8 cup 45 cal.
- Romaine lettuce 1 cup 8 cal.
- Tomato 1 medium 22 cal.
- Salsa ¼ cup 17 cal.

1 orange 45 cal.

Dinner 684
4 oz. of Salmon 240 cal.
1 cup broccoli 30 cal. with 2 teaspoon coconut oil 80 cal.
1 cup baked sweet potato 114 cal. with 1 pat of ghee butter 30 cal.
Functional food 190 cal.

Total 1,671

300-Calorie Meals in About 5 Minutes

See 7SystemsPlan.com for more menus.

Power Shake (270 cal.): functional food, oils, seeds, and vegetables

1. 3 cups spinach 20 cal.
2. 2 tablespoons guacamole 40 cal.
3. 1 tablespoon chia seeds 60 cal.

Blend well, add functional food (150 cal.) and blend briefly

Salmon Melt (342 cal.): grain, protein, dairy, and oil

- 1 slice of whole-grain bread 70 cal.
- 3 oz. canned Alaskan salmon 175 cal. with 1 tablespoon avocado oil mayo 60 cal.
- Tomato 12 cal.
- Cheese 1/4 cup 25 cal.
Broil and enjoy

Fast-Mimicking Diet Menus

FMDs

After your first month on the 7 Systems Plan, try a fast-mimicking diet (FMD). It will take a few weeks for your body to adjust to this, so give it some time. You will be impressed with the results. See 7SystemsPlan.com for more FMD menus.

17-Hour Fast:

Simply use the menus above and change the time you eat to match the following schedule:

- Lunch: 12 p.m.
- Snack: 3 p.m.
- Dinner: 6:30 p.m.

23-Hour Fast:
The 23-hour fast can be used every other day (aggressive), once per week (moderate), or even once per month (easy). Since you are only eating one meal, it is important that it is a good one. I suggest that you use a functional food as part of your meal to insure proper nutrient intake.

5:2 FMD
On two nonconsecutive days per week, restrict your caloric intake to 500 for females and 600 for males. To make this work even better, you can skip breakfast and eat all your food between 12 p.m. and 7 p.m. Again, since you are restricting calories significantly, make sure that you eat well-balanced meals. The addition of a functional food makes this very easy.

Part Seven

Simple At-Home Fitness Test

An easy way to know if you are making progress with your exercise is to do this test each month. Don't forget to record your findings.

If you have health problems, consult your physician before beginning this test.

In one minute, see how many of the following you can do.

- Squats (sit on the edge of a chair and stand up, then go down until you almost touch the chair)
- Push-ups (wall, knee, or toe)
- Sit-ups (bend knees 45 degrees and hook your toes under a couch)

In addition to the exercises above, see how long it takes you to walk or run one mile.

Repeat this test after one month.

Aerobic Exercise Zone

As you become more fit try to keep you heart rate in your aerobic zone. Maximum benefit occurs when are in your zone for 30 minutes per day.

Age	Min-Max Heart Rate (BPM)
15	123 – 164
20	120 – 160
25	117 – 156
30	114 – 152
35	111 – 148
40	108 – 144

Age	Min-Max Heart Rate (BPM)
45	105 – 140
50	102 – 136
55	99 – 132
60	96 – 128
65	90 – 120
70	90 – 120
75	87 – 116

Whole-Body Weight Lifting Interval Routine

This is an easy way to do both an interval training and weight lifting in one 20-minute session. Do 90 seconds of weight lifting (as I describe) followed by a 30-second burst of more intense exercises like jumping jacks, burpees, or running in place.

All you need is a few hand weights. It helps to have light and heavy ones to work the muscles completely. If you are using the correct weight, you should have difficulty completing the last few repetitions of the last set. If it is not that hard, increase the weight next time. You do not build muscles unless you exhaust them.

Lunge Curl

With a weight in each hand, take a step forward with one foot and go down as far as you comfortably can. Come back up, and then do a bicep curl. Step forward with the other leg and repeat. Repeat 10 times.

All lifting should be done slowly. Most of the benefit of this exercise is in the lowering phase, so lower the weight slowly as well.

Squat Press

With a weight in each hand, at shoulder-level, squat down as low as you comfortably can, and then come up. When you are up, press the weights above your head, and then lower them. Repeat 10 times.

Bent Over Curl Fly

With a light weight in each hand, bend forward at a 45-degree angle. Arch your back and keep your head up. Stay in this position while you bring the weight up to your chest, down, and then out to the side. Repeat 10 times.

Push-Ups

You can do push-ups in three ways. The easiest is to stand with your feet a couple of feet from a wall, put your hands on the wall at shoulder height, bend your elbow till you touch the wall with your head, and push away. The second way is to do a push-up on the floor with your knees down. For a regular push-up, keep your back straight with each push. Do 10 if you can, or as many as possible.

Appendix B:
The 7 Systems Plan Online Course

Need more support on your health journey?

While many have had success achieving their health goals with this book, the most successful readers also use the course. Now that you understand your Systems and have an idea of which Systems are sabotaging your health, let this course help you on your journey to get them working for you again.

This groundbreaking content merges the latest health findings in science with simple, practical methods of implementation. You'll receive the tools and support you need to fix your Systems and experience a lifetime of vibrant health.

What you'll learn about:

- All the amazing things the 7 Systems Plan Course can do for you and your loved ones
- The quickest way to make your Systems function optimally for you to have ideal health

- The healthiest and most healing foods that you need to integrate into your diet
- Toxic foods that many people consume every day
- The power of fasting and fast-mimicking diets and practical ways to use them

Here's What Is Included!

Fourteen practical lessons on The 7 Systems, to help you get your Systems working for you fast. These engaging, inspirational, and instructional modules will equip you with the same tools my private patients receive to lose weight, fix their Systems, and regain their health.

When you purchase, you will also get four valuable bonuses!

Bonus 1 – The Maximizing Toolbox

You will get instant access to the tools I give to my patients to help ensure their success.

Bonus 2 – You will get instant access to many power-packed bonus lessons:

- Breaking Food Addiction
- Fasting The Correct Way
- How To Spice Up Your Love Life
- Keys To Making Your Progress Permanent
- The Secrets To Becoming Superhuman
- Making Your Gut Bacteria Work For You
- A Simple Plan To Change Any Behavior
- And Many More

Bonus 3 – You will also get access to the 7 Systems Plan private community:

Got a question for me or a graduate? This is where you get the answers. Get encouragement, meal prep tips, and recipes, and see what successful members are doing.

Bonus 4 – You will get the workbook developed to go with the course.

The 7 Systems Plan Course is for you if...

- You want a coach and guide to help you regain your health.
- You have tried multiple diets and programs, with little to moderate success.
- You have family, friends, or close loved ones who struggle with chronic diseases and you want to help them.
- You are always looking for new, cutting-edge ways to heal your health naturally, without the need for addictive drugs or surgery.
- You want to learn the most up-to-date information on alternative medicine from credible, reliable sources.
- You are confused by all the conflicting health information out there.
- You are curious about how to optimize your Systems to get even healthier.
- You have done everything everyone tells you, but you still aren't seeing results.
- You are looking for a natural approach to help with obesity, heart disease, diabetes, or autoimmune diseases.
- You want to get healthy so your doctor will take you off prescriptions
- You just want to feel good again.

So, if this sounds like you, join the countless men and women around the world who have committed to changing their lives using the 7 Systems Plan course. Now is your time to make that much-needed transformation and get the results you deserve.

Why we know you'll love it:

This a very cost-effective way to create a lifestyle of health trans-formation and lasting weight loss.

What people are saying:

- "So far, I have lost 51 pounds, and my insulin, glucose, and resting heart rate are in the excellent category!" —Jody
- "I feel better about myself, and my weight loss (45 pounds) is noticed by my family, and they are encouraged to try it for themselves." —Chris
- "I have lost almost 35 pounds and love how I feel. I haven't felt this good in 30 years!" —Carrie
- "The 7 Systems Plan has not just shown me *how* to lose weight, but *why* my body's Systems work together and how I can optimize my life to enhance these natural Systems." —Tom
- "I have lost 17 pounds and have much more energy. More than I had years ago." —Patty
- "I enjoy eating all my 1,300 calories for the day in a 7-hour window. Because then I am satisfied and can go without eating for another 17 hours." —Sheila

Ready to get started? Visit 7SystemsPlan.com today!

Index

Endnotes

Chapter 1

1. Maffetone, Philip B., Ivan Rivera-Dominguez, and Paul B. Laursen. "Overfat and Underfat: New Terms and Definitions Long Overdue." *Frontiers in Public Health* 4 (2017). doi:10.3389/fpubh.2016.00279.

   "Deeper than Obesity: A majority of people is now overfat." *ScienceDaily*. January 3, 2017. https://www.sciencedaily.com/releases/2017/01/170103122342.htm.

   "Fat and getting fatter: U.S. obesity rates to soar by 2030." *Reuters*. September 18, 2012. http://www.reuters.com/article/us-obesity-us-idUSBRE88H0RA20120918.

2. Fothergill, Erin, Juen Guo, Lilian Howard, Jennifer C. Kerns, Nicolas D. Knuth, Robert Brychta, Kong Y. Chen, Monica C. Skarulis, Mary Walter, Peter J. Walter, and Kevin D. Hall. "Persistent metabolic adaptation 6 years after "The Biggest Loser" competition." *Obesity* 24, no. 8 (2016): 1612-619. doi:10.1002/oby.21538.

3. Johnell, O., and J. A. Kanis. "An estimate of the worldwide prevalence and disability associated with osteoporotic fractures." Osteoporosis

International 17, no. 12 (2006): 1726-733. doi:10.1007/s00198-006-0172-4.

4. Ahmed, Dr. Murtaza, Marjorie Campbell Says, Dr. Mustafa Ahmed, and Dr. Jason L. Guichard, MD, PhD. "Sarcopenia – Age Related Muscle Loss." *MyHeart*. August 02, 2015. https://myheart.net/articles/sarcopenia-age-related-muscle-loss/.

5. Masters, Ryan K., Eric N. Reither, Daniel A. Powers, Y. Claire Yang, Andrew E. Burger, and Bruce G. Link. "The Impact of Obesity on US Mortality Levels: The Importance of Age and Cohort Factors in Population Estimates." *American Journal of Public Health* 103, no. 10 (2013): 1895-901. doi:10.2105/ajph.2013.301379.

6. Cooper, Cyrus, Elizabeth J. Atkinson, Steven J. Jacobsen, W. Michael O'Fallon, and L. Joseph Melton. "Population-Based Study of Survival after Osteoporotic Fractures." *American Journal of Epidemiology* 137, no. 9 (1993): 1001-005. doi:10.1093/oxfordjournals.aje.a116756.

7. Leibson, Cynthia L., Anna N. A. Tosteson, Sherine E. Gabriel, Jeanine E. Ransom, and L. Joseph Melton. "Mortality, Disability, and Nursing Home Use for Persons with and without Hip Fracture: A Population-Based Study." *Journal of the American Geriatrics Society* 50, no. 10 (2002): 1644-650. doi:10.1046/j.1532-5415.2002.50455.x.

   Magaziner, J., E. M. Simonsick, T. M. Kashner, J. R. Hebel, and J. E. Kenzora. "Predictors of Functional Recovery One Year Following Hospital Discharge for Hip Fracture: A Prospective Study." *Journal of Gerontology* 45, no. 3 (1990). doi:10.1093/geronj/45.3.m101.

   Riggs, B.l., and L.j. Melton. "The worldwide problem of osteoporosis: Insights afforded by epidemiology." *Bone* 17, no. 5 (1995). doi: 10.1016/8756-3282(95)00258-4.

   Kannus, Pekka. "Epidemiology of Osteoporotic Ankle Fractures in Elderly Persons in Finland." *Annals of Internal Medicine* 125, no. 12 (1996): 975. doi:10.7326/0003-4819-125-12-199612150-00007.

8. Rome, Peter L. "Neurovertebral influence upon the autonomic nervous system: some of the somato-autonomic evidence to date." *Chiropractic Journal of Australia* 39, no. 1 (March 2009).

   http://www.chiroindex.org/wp-content/uploads/2010/11/Rome_PL_2009.pdf.

9. Buettner, Dan. "How to Live to be 100+," TED video, filmed September 2009,

   https://www.ted.com/talks/dan_buettner_how_to_live_to_be_100.

10. Archer, Edward, Gregory A. Hand, and Steven N. Blair. "Validity of U.S. Nutritional Surveillance: National Health and Nutrition Examination Survey Caloric Energy Intake Data, 1971–2010." *PLOS ONE*. http:// journals.plos.org/plosone/article?id=10.1371%2Fannotation%2Fc313df 3a-52bd-4cbe-af14-6676480d1a43.

11. Fryar, Cheryl D., M.S.P.H., Margaret D. Carroll, M.S.P.H., and Cynthia L. Ogden, PhD, Division of Health and Nutrition Examination Surveys. "Prevalence of Overweight, Obesity, and Extreme Obesity Among Adults: United States, 1960–1962 Through 2011–2012." *Centers for Disease Control and Prevention.* (September 19, 2014) https://www.cdc. gov/nchs/data/hestat/obesity_adult_11_12/obesity_adult_11_12.htm.

    Murray, Christopher J. L. "The State of US Health, 1990-2010." *JAMA: The Journal of the American Medical Association* 310, no. 6 (2013): 591. doi:10.1001/jama.2013.13805.

12. Whitehead, Ross D., Gozde Ozakinci, Ian D. Stephen, and David I. Perrett. "Appealing to Vanity: Could Potential Appearance Improvement Motivate Fruit and Vegetable Consumption?" *American Journal of Public Health* 102, no. 2 (2012): 207-11. doi:10.2105/ajph.2011.300405.

13. Blanchflower, David, Andrew Oswald, and Sarah Stewart-Brown. "Is Psychological Well-being Linked to the Consumption of Fruit and Vegetables?" *Andrew Oswald.* (2012) http://www.andrewoswald.com/ docs/October2FruitAndVeg2012BlanchOswaldStewartBrown.pdf

14. Estruch, Ramón, Emilio Ros, Jordi Salas-Salvadó, Maria-Isabel Covas, Dolores Corella, Fernando Arós, Enrique Gómez-Gracia, Valentina Ruiz-Gutiérrez, Miquel Fiol, José Lapetra, Rosa Maria Lamuela-Raventos, Lluís Serra-Majem, Xavier Pintó, Josep Basora, Miguel Angel Muñoz, José V. Sorlí, José Alfredo Martínez, and Miguel Angel Martínez-González. "Primary Prevention of Cardiovascular Disease with a Mediterranean Diet." *New England Journal of Medicine* 368, no. 14 (2013): 1279-290. doi:10.1056/nejmoa1200303.

15. Brandhorst, Sebastian, In Young Choi, Min Wei, Chia Wei Cheng, Sargis Sedrakyan, Gerardo Navarrete, Louis Dubeau, Li Peng Yap, Ryan Park, Manlio Vinciguerra, Stefano Di Biase, Hamed Mirzaei, Mario G. Mirisola, Patra Childress, Lingyun Ji, Susan Groshen, Fabio Penna, Patrizio Odetti, Laura Perin, Peter S. Conti, Yuji Ikeno, Brian K. Kennedy, Pinchas Cohen, Todd E. Morgan, Tanya B. Dorff, and Valter D. Longo. "A Periodic Diet that Mimics Fasting Promotes Multi-System Regeneration, Enhanced Cognitive Performance, and Healthspan." *Cell Metabolism* 22, no. 1 (2015): 86-99. doi:10.1016/j.cmet.2015.05.012.

Chapter 2

1. National Institutes of Health, U.S. Department of Health and Human Services. "Opportunities and Challenges in Digestive Diseases Research: Recommendations of the National Commission on Digestive Diseases." National Institutes of Health; 2009. NIH Publication 08–6514.

2. *The Sensitive Gut*. Report. Harvard Medical School. 2017. https://www.health.harvard.edu/promotions/harvard-health-publications/the-sensitive-gut.

3. "Digestive problems are one of the top issues that send people to their doctors"

4. Schmidt, Charles. "Mental Health May Depend on Creatures in the Gut." *Scientific American*. March 1, 2015. https://www.scientificamerican.com/article/mental-health-may-depend-on-creatures-in-the-gut/.

5. Pray, Leslie A. *Relationships among the brain, the digestive system, and eating behavior: workshop summary*. Washington, D.C.: The National Academies Press, 2015.

6. Robinson, E., P. Aveyard, A. Daley, K. Jolly, A. Lewis, D. Lycett, and S. Higgs. "Eating attentively: a systematic review and meta-analysis of the effect of food intake memory and awareness on eating." *American Journal of Clinical Nutrition* 97, no. 4 (2013): 728-42. doi:10.3945/ajcn.112.045245.

7. Gomm, Willy, Klaus Von Holt, Friederike Thomé, Karl Broich, Wolfgang Maier, Anne Fink, Gabriele Doblhammer, and Britta Haenisch. "Association of Proton Pump Inhibitors With Risk of Dementia." *JAMA Neurology* 73, no. 4 (2016): 410. doi:10.1001/jamaneurol.2015.4791.

8. Goldstein, Jay, and Byron Cryer. "Gastrointestinal injury associated with NSAID use: a case study and review of risk factors and preventative strategies." *Drug, Healthcare and Patient Safety*, January 22, 2015, 31. doi:10.2147/dhps.s71976.

9. Metchnikoff, Elie, and Chalmers, Mitchell P. *Prolongation of life: optimistic studies*. New York & London: G.P. Putnam's Sons, 1908. You can find the entire book archived: https://archive.org/details/prolongationof li00metciala.

10. Abou-Donia, Mohamed B., Eman M. El-Masry, Ali A. Abdel-Rahman, Roger E. Mclendon, and Susan S. Schiffman. "Splenda Alters Gut Microflora and Increases Intestinal P-Glycoprotein and Cytochrome P-450 in Male Rats." *Journal of Toxicology and Environmental Health*, Part A 71, no. 21 (2008): 1415-429. doi:10.1080/15287390802328630.

11. *Guidelines for the Evaluation of Probiotics in Food.* PDF. Food and Agriculture Organization (FAO) and World Health Organization (WHO), May 1, 2002.
    http://www.who.int/foodsafety/fs_management/en/probiotic_guidelines.pdf

12. Stenman, Lotta K., Markus J. Lehtinen, Nils Meland, Jeffrey E. Christensen, Nicolas Yeung, Markku T. Saarinen, Michael Courtney, Rémy Burcelin, Marja-Leena Lähdeaho, Jüri Linros, Dan Apter, Mika Scheinin, Hilde Kloster Smerud, Aila Rissanen, and Sampo Lahtinen. "Probiotic With or Without Fiber Controls Body Fat Mass, Associated With Serum Zonulin, in Overweight and Obese Adults—Randomized Controlled Trial." *EBioMedicine* 13 (August 2016): 190-200. doi:10.1016/j.ebiom.2016.10.036.

13. "UltraBiotic Integrity* - †Based on a six-month clinical study of overweight individuals taking Bifidobacterium animalis lactis B-420™ as compared to placebo (Stenman LK, et al. EBioMedicine. 2016;13:190-200.)

14. Ridaura, V. K., J. J. Faith, F. E. Rey, J. Cheng, A. E. Duncan, A. L. Kau, N. W. Griffin, V. Lombard, B. Henrissat, J. R. Bain, M. J. Muehlbauer, O. Ilkayeva, C. F. Semenkovich, K. Funai, D. K. Hayashi, B. J. Lyle, M. C. Martini, L. K. Ursell, J. C. Clemente, W. Van Treuren, W. A. Walters, R. Knight, C. B. Newgard, A. C. Heath, and J. I. Gordon. "Gut Microbiota from Twins Discordant for Obesity Modulate Metabolism in Mice." *Science* 341, no. 6150 (2013): 1241214. doi:10.1126/science.1241214.

Chapter 3

1. Mozaffarian, Dariush, Emelia J. Benjamin, Alan S. Go, Donna K. Arnett, Michael J. Blaha, Mary Cushman, Sarah De Ferranti, Jean-Pierre Després, Heather J. Fullerton, Virginia J. Howard, Mark D. Huffman, Suzanne E. Judd, Brett M. Kissela, Daniel T. Lackland, Judith H. Lichtman, Lynda D. Lisabeth, Simin Liu, Rachel H. Mackey, David B. Matchar, Darren K. Mcguire, Emile R. Mohler, Claudia S. Moy, Paul Muntner, Michael E. Mussolino, Khurram Nasir, Robert W. Neumar, Graham Nichol, Latha Palaniappan, Dilip K. Pandey, Mathew J. Reeves, Carlos J. Rodriguez, Paul D. Sorlie, Joel Stein, Amytis Towfighi, Tanya N. Turan, Salim S. Virani, Joshua Z. Willey, Daniel Woo, Robert W. Yeh, and Melanie B. Turner. "Heart Disease and Stroke Statistics—2015 Update." *Circulation* 131, no. 4 (2014). doi:10.1161/cir.0000000000000152.

2. "Heart Disease Facts." The Heart Foundation. https://www.theheart-foundation.org/heart-disease-facts/heart-disease-statistics/.

3. "Diabetes Has Become One of the Most Lethal Diseases in the World." *Mercola.com*. Accessed February 22, 2017. http://articles.mercola.com/sites/articles/archive/2017/02/22/diabetes-expensive-lethal-disease.aspx.

4. Sanchez, Janine, M.D. "Type 2 diabetes becoming a childhood epidemic." *Miamiherald.com*. November 1, 2016. http://www.miamiherald.com/living/health-fitness/article111778712.html.

5. Greger, Michael, M.D., FACLM. "Heart Disease Starts in Childhood." *NutritionFacts.org*. September 23, 2013. https://nutritionfacts.org/video/heart-disease-starts-in-childhood/.

6. Vogel, Robert A., Mary C. Corretti, and Gary D. Plotnick. "Effect of a Single High-Fat Meal on Endothelial Function in Healthy Subjects." *The American Journal of Cardiology* 79, no. 3 (1997): 350-54. doi:10.1016/s0002-9149(96)00760-6.

7. Raji, Cyrus A., Kirk I. Erickson, Oscar L. Lopez, Lewis H. Kuller, H. Michael Gach, Paul M. Thompson, Mario Riverol, and James T. Becker. "Regular Fish Consumption and Age-Related Brain Gray Matter Loss." *American Journal of Preventive Medicine* 47, no. 4 (July 29, 2014): 444-51. doi: 10.1016/j.amepre.2014.05.037.

8. Whalley, Lawrence J., Helen C. Fox, Klaus W. Wahle, and And John M Starr. "Cognitive aging, childhood intelligence, and the use of food supplements: possible involvement of n-3 fatty acids." *The American Journal of Clinical Nutrition*. December 2004, vol. 80, no. 6 1650-1657. http://ajcn.nutrition.org/content/80/6/1650.full#abstract-1.

9. Michels, Karin B., Bernard A. Rosner, Wm. Cameron Chumlea, Graham A. Colditz, and Walter C. Willett. "Preschool diet and adult risk of breast cancer." *International Journal of Cancer* 118, no. 3 (2005): 749-54. doi:10.1002/ijc.21407.

10. Roizen, Michael, MD. "How many people take statin drugs? - Cardiovascular Agent." *Sharecare*. https://www.sharecare.com/health/cardiovascular-drugs/how-many-people-take-statin.

11. Studer, Marco, Matthias Briel, Bernd Leimenstoll, Tracy R. Glass, and Heiner C. Bucher. "Effect of Different Antilipidemic Agents and Diets on Mortality." *Archives of Internal Medicine* 165, no. 7 (2005): 725. doi:10.1001/archinte.165.7.725.

12. Golomb, Beatrice A., and Marcella A. Evans. "Statin Adverse Effects." *American Journal of Cardiovascular Drugs* 8, no. 6 (2008): 373-418. doi:10.2165/0129784-200808060-00004.

13. Dobberstein, Linda J. "Statin Drugs Cause Atherosclerosis and Heart Failure." *Wellness Resources.* February 6, 2015. http://www.wellness resources.com/health/articles/statin_drugs_stimulate_atherosclerosis_ and_heart_failure/.

14. Allen, N. E., P. N. Appleby, G. K. Davey, R. Kaaks, S. Rinaldi, and T. J. Key. "The associations of diet with serum insulin-like growth factor I and its main binding proteins in 292 women meat-eaters, vegetarians, and vegans." *Cancer Epidemiology, Biomarkers & Prevention: a publication of the American Association for Cancer Research, cosponsored by the American Society of Preventive Oncology.* November 2002. https://www.ncbi.nlm. nih.gov/pubmed/12433724.

15. Gholipour, Bahar. "Diet High in Meat Proteins Raises Cancer Risk for Middle-Aged People." *Scientific American.* March 4, 2014. https:// www.scientificamerican.com/article/diet-high-in-meat-proteins-raises- cancer-risk-for-middle-aged-people/.

16. Van, E., F. A. Hospers, G. Navis, M. F. Engberink, E. J. Brink, J. M. Geleijnse, M. A. Van, R. O. Gans, and S. J. Bakker. "Dietary acid load and rapid progression to end-stage renal disease of diabetic nephropathy in Westernized South Asian people." *Journal of Nephrology.* Jan. & Feb. 2011. https://www.ncbi.nlm.nih.gov/pubmed/20872351.

17. Reinagel, Monica. "How Much Protein Can the Body Absorb?" Scientific American. April 23, 2014. Accessed August 21, 2017. https://www. scientificamerican.com/article/how-much-protein-can-the-body- absorb/.

18. Kern, Fred. "Normal Plasma Cholesterol in an 88-Year-Old Man Who Eats 25 Eggs a Day." *New England Journal of Medicine* 324, no. 13 (1991): 896-99. doi:10.1056/nejm199103283241306.

19. Bao, Ying, Jiali Han, Frank B. Hu, Edward L. Giovannucci, Meir J. Stampfer, Walter C. Willett, and Charles S. Fuchs. "Association of Nut Consumption with Total and Cause-Specific Mortality." *New England Journal of Medicine* 369, no. 21 (2013): 2001-011. doi:10.1056/ nejmoa1307352.

20. Wien, M. A., J. M. Sabaté, D. N. Iklé, S. E. Cole, and F. R. Kandeel. "Almonds vs complex carbohydrates in a weight reduction program." *International Journal of Obesity* 27, no. 11 (2003): 1365-372. doi:10.1038/ sj.ijo.0802411.

21. Ros, Emilio. "Health Benefits of Nut Consumption." *Nutrients* 2, no. 7 (2010): 652-82. doi:10.3390/nu2070652.

22. Joslin Diabetes Center. "Asian Americans & Diabetes." *Joslin Diabetes Center.* http://www.joslin.org/info/Asian_Americans_and_Diabetes.html.

23. Bray, George A., Samara Joy Nielsen. "Consumption of high-fructose corn syrup in beverages may play a role in the epidemic of obesity." *The American Journal of Clinical Nutrition.* April 01, 2004. http://ajcn.nutrition. org/content/79/4/537.long.

24. Pase, Matthew P., Jayandra J. Himali, Alexa S. Beiser, Hugo J. Aparicio, Claudia L. Satizabal, Ramachandran S. Vasan, Sudha Seshadri, and Paul F. Jacques. "Sugar- and Artificially Sweetened Beverages and the Risks of Incident Stroke and Dementia: A Prospective Cohort Study." Stroke. January 01, 2017. http://stroke.ahajournals.org/content/ early/2017/04/20/STROKEAHA.116.016027

25. Ludwig, D. S., J. A. Majzoub, A. Al-Zahrani, G. E. Dallal, I. Blanco, and S. B. Roberts. "High Glycemic Index Foods, Overeating, and Obesity." *Pediatrics* 103, no. 3 (1999). doi:10.1542/peds.103.3.e26.

26. Mercola, Joseph, DO. "Are bagels and breakfast cereal as bad as cigarettes? Report shows they can raise risk of lung cancer by 49%!" *Mercola. com.* http://articles.mercola.com/sites/articles/archive/2016/03/23/ultra-processed-foods.aspx.

27. Carr, C. Jelleff, and R.f. Shangraw. "Nutritional and Pharmaceutical Aspects of Calcium Supplementation." *American Pharmacy* 27, no. 2 (1987): 49-56. doi:10.1016/s0160-3450(15)32077-8.

28. Jones, Jennifer L., Maria Luz Fernandez, Mark S. Mcintosh, Wadie Najm, Mariana C. Calle, Colleen Kalynych, Clare Vukich, Jacqueline Barona, Daniela Ackermann, Jung Eun Kim, Vivek Kumar, Michelle Lott, Jeff S. Volek, and Robert H. Lerman. "A Mediterranean-style low-glycemic-load diet improves variables of metabolic syndrome in women, and addition of a phytochemical-rich functional food enhances benefits on lipoprotein metabolism." *Journal of Clinical Lipidology* 5, no. 3 (2011): 188-96. doi:10.1016/j.jacl.2011.03.002.

29. Leblanc, Erin S., Joanne H. Rizzo, Kathryn L. Pedula, Kristine E. Ensrud, Jane Cauley, Marc Hochberg, and Teresa A. Hillier. "Associations Between 25-Hydroxyvitamin D and Weight Gain in Elderly Women." *Journal of Women's Health* 21, no. 10 (October 2012): 1066-073. doi:10.1089/jwh.2012.3506.

31. Kennel, Kurt A., Matthew T. Drake, and Daniel L. Hurley. "Vitamin D Deficiency in Adults: When to Test and How to Treat." *Mayo Clinic Proceedings* 85, no. 8 (2010): 752-58. doi:10.4065/mcp.2010.0138.

32. Thacher, Tom D., and Bart L. Clarke. "Vitamin D Insufficiency." *Mayo Clinic Proceedings* 86, no. 1 (2011): 50-60. doi:10.4065/mcp.2010.0567.

33. Scragg, Robert, Rodney Jackson, Ian M. Holdaway, Thomas Lim, and Robert Beaglehole. "Myocardial Infarction is Inversely Associated with

Plasma 25-Hydroxyvitamin D3 Levels: A Community-Based Study." *International Journal of Epidemiology* 19, no. 3 (September 19, 1990): 559-63. doi:10.1093/ije/19.3.559.

34. Krause, Rolfdieter, Malte Bühring, Werner Hopfenmüller, Michael F. Holick, and Arya M. Sharma. "Ultraviolet B and blood pressure." *The Lancet* 352, no. 9129 (August 29, 1998): 709-10. doi:10.1016/s0140-6736(05)60827-6.

35. Chiu, K. C., A. Chu, V. L. Go, and M. F. Saad. "Hypovitaminosis D is associated with insulin resistance and beta cell dysfunction." *The American Journal of Clinical Nutrition*. May 2004. https://www.ncbi.nlm.nih.gov/pubmed/15113720.

36. Bjelakovic, G., L. Gluud, D. Nikolova, K. Whitfield, J. Wetterslev, RG Simonetti, M. Bjelakovic, and C. Gluud. "Vitamin D supplementation for prevention of mortality in adults." *Cochrane.org*. January 10, 2014. http://www.cochrane.org/CD007470/ENDOC_vitamin-d-supplementation-for-prevention-of-mortality-in-adults.

37. Siscovick, David S. "Dietary Intake and Cell Membrane Levels of Long-Chain n-3 Polyunsaturated Fatty Acids and the Risk of Primary Cardiac Arrest." *JAMA: The Journal of the American Medical Association* 274, no. 17 (1995): 1363. doi:10.1001/jama.1995.03530170043030.

38. Morris, Martha Clare, Denis A. Evans, Julia L. Bienias, Christine C. Tangney, David A. Bennett, Robert S. Wilson, Neelum Aggarwal, and Julie Schneider. "Consumption of Fish and n-3 Fatty Acids and Risk of Incident Alzheimer Disease." *Archives of Neurology* 60, no. 7 (2003): 940. doi:10.1001/archneur.60.7.940.

Chapter 4

1. Rosenthal, Thomas C., Barbara A. Majeroni, Richard Pretorious, and Khalid Malik. "Fatigue: An Overview." American Family Physician. November 15, 2008. http://www.aafp.org/afp/2008/1115/p1173.html.

2. Litchy, Andrew P., ND. "Mitochondrial Dysfunction: A Cause and Symptom of Chronic Illness." *Bhakti Wellness Center BLOG*. June 14, 2016. http://bhakticlinic.com/blog/mitochondrial-dysfunction-a-cause-and-symptom-of-chronic-illness/.

3. Seyfried, Thomas N. "Cancer as a mitochondrial metabolic disease." *Frontiers in Cell and Developmental Biology* 3 (2015). doi:10.3389/fcell.2015.00043.

4. Nigam, Anil, Dr., and University of Montreal. "Study: Every junk food meal damages your arteries!" *Sherman Heart & Vascular Blog*. November

02, 2012. Accessed July 28, 2017. https://shermanheart.wordpress.com/2012/10/31/study-every-junk-food-meal-damages-your-arteries/.

5. Shandwick, Weber. "Americans with 'phytonutrient gap' fall short in nutrients that may support immune health." *EurekAlert*. October 28, 2010. https://www.eurekalert.org/pub_releases/2010-10/wsw-aw102710.php.

6. He, Feng J., Caryl A. Nowson, and Graham A. Macgregor. "Fruit and vegetable consumption and stroke: meta-analysis of cohort studies." The Lancet 367, no. 9507 (January 28, 2006): 320-26. doi:10.1016/s0140-6736(06)68069-0.

7. Nutrilite. "America's Phytonutrient Report 2009 Releases Revised Analysis." New Hope Network. February 7, 2010. America's Phytonutrient Report Releases Revised Analysis. http://www.newhope.com/supply-news-amp-analysis/americas-phytonutrient-report-releases-revised-analysis

8. Jaslow, Ryan. "CDC: 80 percent of American adults don't get recommended exercise." *CBS News*. May 03, 2013. Accessed July 28, 2017. http://www.cbsnews.com/news/cdc-80-percent-of-american-adults-dont-get-recommended-exercise/.

9. Lee, I-Min, Eric J. Shiroma, Felipe Lobelo, Pekka Puska, Steven N. Blair, and Peter T. Katzmarzyk. "Effect of physical inactivity on major non-communicable diseases worldwide: an analysis of burden of disease and life expectancy." *The Lancet* 380, no. 9838 (July 18, 2012): 219-29. doi:10.1016/s0140-6736(12)61031-9.

10. Ladenvall, Per, Carina U. Persson, Zacharias Mandalenakis, Lars Wilhelmsen, Gunnar Grimby, Kurt Svärdsudd, and Per-Olof Hansson. "Low aerobic capacity in middle-aged men associated with increased mortality rates during 45 years of follow-up." *European Journal of Preventive Cardiology* 23, no. 14 (2016): 1557-564. doi:10.1177/2047487316655466.

11. Robinson, Matthew M., Surendra Dasari, Adam R. Konopka, Matthew L. Johnson, S. Manjunatha, Raul Ruiz Esponda, Rickey E. Carter, Ian R. Lanza, and K. Sreekumaran Nair. "Enhanced Protein Translation Underlies Improved Metabolic and Physical Adaptations to Different Exercise Training Modes in Young and Old Humans." *Cell Metabolism* 25, no. 3 (March 7, 2017): 581-92. doi:10.1016/j.cmet.2017.02.009.

12. Hambrecht, R. "Percutaneous Coronary Angioplasty Compared With Exercise Training in Patients With Stable Coronary Artery Disease: A Randomized Trial." *Circulation* 109, no. 11 (2004): 1371-378. doi: 10.1161/01.cir.0000121360.31954.1f.

13. Wen, Chi Pang, Jackson Pui Man Wai, Min Kuang Tsai, Yi Chen Yang, Ting Yuan David Cheng, Meng-Chih Lee, Hui Ting Chan, Chwen

Keng Tsao, Shan Pou Tsai, and Xifeng Wu. "Minimum amount of physical activity for reduced mortality and extended life expectancy: a prospective cohort study." *The Lancet* 378, no. 9798 (2011): 1244-253. doi:10.1016/s0140-6736(11)60749-6.

14. Hayashi, Tomoshige, Kei Tsumura, Chika Suematsu, Kunio Okada, Satoru Fujii, and Ginji Endo. "Walking to Work and the Risk for Hypertension in Men: The Osaka Health Survey." *Annals of Internal Medicine* 131, no. 1 (1999): 21. doi:10.7326/0003-4819-131-1-199907060-00005.

15. Moore, Steven C., I-Min Lee, Elisabete Weiderpass, Peter T. Campbell, Joshua N. Sampson, Cari M. Kitahara, Sarah K. Keadle, Hannah Arem, Amy Berrington de Gonzalez, Patricia Hartge, Hans-Olov Adami, Cindy K. Blair, Kristin B. Borch, Eric Boyd, David P. Check, Agnès Fournier, Neal D. Freedman, Marc Gunter, Mattias Johannson, Kay-Tee Khaw, MsC, Martha S. Linet, Nicola Orsini, Yikyung Park, Elio Riboli, Kim Robien, Catherine Schairer, Howard Sesso, Michael Spriggs, Roy Van Dusen, Alicja Wolk, Charles E. Matthews, Alpa V. Patel. "Association of Leisure-Time Physical Activity With Risk of 26 Types of Cancer in 1.44 Million Adults." *JAMA Internal Medicine* 2016; 176(6):816-825.

16. Zhang, Yuan, Chao Xie, Hai Wang, Robin M. Foss, Morgan Clare, Eva Vertes George, Shiwu Li, Adam Katz, Henrique Cheng, Yousong Ding, Dongqi Tang, Westley H. Reeves, and Li-Jun Yang. "Irisin exerts dual effects on browning and adipogenesis of human white adipocytes." *American Journal of Physiology - Endocrinology and Metabolism* 311, no. 2 (2016). doi:10.1152/ajpendo.00094.2016.

17. Cell, Press. "How exercise—interval training in particular—helps your mitochondria stave off old age." ScienceDaily. March 7, 2017. https://www.sciencedaily.com/releases/2017/03/170307155214.htm.

18. Little, Jonathan P., Adeel Safdar, Carley R. Benton, and David C. Wright. "Skeletal muscle and beyond: the role of exercise as a mediator of systemic mitochondrial biogenesis." *Applied Physiology, Nutrition, and Metabolism* 36, no. 5 (2011): 598-607. doi:10.1139/h11-076.

19. Trapp, E. G., D. J. Chisholm, J. Freund, and S. H. Boutcher. "The effects of high-intensity intermittent exercise training on fat loss and fasting insulin levels of young women." *International Journal of Obesity* 32, no. 4 (2008): 684-91. doi:10.1038/sj.ijo.0803781.

20. Heydari, M., J. Freund, and S. H. Boutcher. "The Effect of High-Intensity Intermittent Exercise on Body Composition of Overweight Young Males." *Journal of Obesity* 2012 (March 2012): 1-8. doi:10.1155/2012/480467.

21. Stokes, K.a., M.e. Nevill, G.m. Hall, and H.k.a. Lakomy. "The time course of the human growth hormone response to a 6 s and a 30 s cycle

ergometer sprint." *Journal of Sports Sciences* 20, no. 6 (2002): 487-94. doi:10.1080/02640410252925152.

22. Bravata, Dena M., Crystal Smith-Spangler, Vandana Sundaram, Allison L. Gienger, Nancy Lin, Robyn Lewis, Christopher D. Stave, Ingram Olkin, and John R. Sirard. "Using Pedometers to Increase Physical Activity and Improve Health." *JAMA: The Journal of the American Medical Association* 298, no. 19 (2007): 2296. doi:10.1001/jama.298.19.2296.

23. White, James R., David A. Case, D. Mcwhirter, and A. M. Mattison. "Enhanced sexual behavior in exercising men." *Archives of Sexual Behavior* 19, no. 3 (1990): 193-209. doi:10.1007/bf01541546.

24. Smith, G. D., S. Frankel, and J. Yarnell. "Sex and death: are they related? Findings from the Caerphilly cohort study." *BMJ* 315, no. 7123 (1997): 1641-644. doi:10.1136/bmj.315.7123.1641.

25. Weeks, David, Jamie James. *Secrets of the Superyoung: The Scientific Reasons Some People Look Ten Years Younger Than They Really Are—and How You Can, Too*. New York City: Berkley Books, 1999.

Chapter 5

1. Araujo, Andre B., Gretchen R. Esche, Varant Kupelian, Amy B. O'Donnell, Thomas G. Travison, Rachel E. Williams, Richard V. Clark, and John B. Mckinlay. "Prevalence of Symptomatic Androgen Deficiency in Men." *The Journal of Clinical Endocrinology & Metabolism* 92, no. 11 (2007): 4241-247. doi:10.1210/jc.2007-1245.

2. "Prevalence and Impact of Thyroid Disease." *American Thyroid Association*. Accessed June 01, 2017. https://www.thyroid.org/media-main/about-hypothyroidism/.

3. Roden, M., T. B. Price, G. Perseghin, K. F. Petersen, D. L. Rothman, G. W. Cline, and G. I. Shulman. "Mechanism of free fatty acid-induced insulin resistance in humans." *Journal of Clinical Investigation* 97, no. 12 (1996): 2859-865. doi:10.1172/jci118742.

4. Hartz-Seeley, Deborah S. "Chronic stress is linked to the six leading causes of death." *Miami Herald*. March 21, 2014. http://www.miamiherald.com/living/article1961770.html.

5. Heminway, John, director. *Stress: Portrait of a Killer*. National Geographic Television, 2008.

6. O'Brien, Jennifer. "UCSF-led study suggests link between psychological stress and cell aging." *UC San Francisco*. November 29, 2004. https://www.ucsf.edu/news/2004/11/5230/ucsf-led-study-suggests-link-between-psychological-stress-and-cell-aging.

7. Gopinath, B., A. E. Buyken, V. M. Flood, M. Empson, E. Rochtchina, and P. Mitchell. "Consumption of polyunsaturated fatty acids, fish, and nuts and risk of inflammatory disease mortality." *American Journal of Clinical Nutrition* 93, no. 5 (2011): 1073-079. doi:10.3945/ajcn.110.009977.

8. Alderman, Lesley. "Breathe. Exhale. Repeat: The Benefits of Controlled Breathing." *The New York Times*. November 09, 2016. https://www.nytimes.com/2016/11/09/well/mind/breathe-exhale-repeat-the-benefits-of-controlled-breathing.html?_r=0.

9. Twal, Waleed O., Amy E. Wahlquist, and Sundaravadivel Balasubramanian. "Yogic breathing when compared to attention control reduces the levels of pro-inflammatory biomarkers in saliva: a pilot randomized controlled trial." *BMC Complementary and Alternative Medicine* 16, no. 1 (2016). doi:10.1186/s12906-016-1286-7.

10. Shomon, Mary. "An Overview of Thyroid Disease." *Verywell*. July 27, 2016. https://www.verywell.com/thyroid-4014636.

11. Heger, Marianne, Boris M. Ventskovskiy, Irina Borzenko, Kyra C. Kneis, Reinhard Rettenberger, Marietta Kaszkin-Bettag, and Peter W. Heger. "Efficacy and safety of a special extract of Rheum rhaponticum (ERr 731) in perimenopausal women with climacteric complaints." *Menopause* 13, no. 5 (Sept. & Oct. 2006): 744-59. doi:10.1097/01.gme. 0000240632.08182.e4.

12. Hormone Replacement Therapy (HRT) was very popular until the women's health study was done in 2002. During the study, they found that using synthetic hormones caused an increase in heart attack, stroke, blood clots, and breast cancer.

The dangers were found only in women who began hormone replacement therapy after age 60. Since that time, it has been found that these findings were often distorted, oversimplified, or wrong. There is a time and place for HRT, and it can be done safely.

However, I believe that a much safer way is to use hormones that are identical to the ones your body produces. They are not drugs, are not synthetic, and are available at compounding pharmacies. They have been used safely for decades and can be very helpful to some women, especially if they have had their ovaries or uterus removed.

It is very important to have a test done before any type of treatment is begun. Hormone levels can vary from one woman to another by 200% to 1,500%. Hormones can be taken in pills, creams, or by transmucosal (vaginal) administration. I believe the most beneficial way for most women is transmucosal. A general rule is to use the lowest dose you can to fix the problems.

Source: Harvard Health. "Bioidentical hormones: Help or hype?" *Harvard Health Publications*. September 2011. https://www.health.harvard.edu/womens-health/bioidentical-hormones-help-or-hype.

13. McCoy, Matthew. "Evaluation of a Standardized Wellness Protocol to Improve Anthropometric and Physiologic Function and to Reduce Health Risk Factors: A Retrospective Analysis of Outcome." *The Journal of Alternative and Complementary Medicine* 17, no. 1 (January 11, 2011): 39-44. doi:10.1089/acm.2010.0113.

14. Rome, Peter L. "Neurovertebral Influence Upon the Autonomic Nervous System: Some of The Somato-Autonomic Evidence To Date." *Chiropractic Journal of Australia* 39, no. 1 (March 2009). http://www.chiroindex.org/wp-content/uploads/2010/11/Rome_PL_2009.pdf.

15. Bitenieks, Madars. "Health benefits of chiropractic care for asymptomatic persons." *Chiropractic Leadership Alliance*. June 01, 2004. http://www.subluxation.com/health-benefits-of-chiropractic-care-for-asymptomatic-persons/.

16. Zhang, John, Douglas Dean, Dennis Nosco, Dennis Strathopulos, and Minas Floros. "Effect of Chiropractic Care on Heart Rate Variability and Pain in a Multisite Clinical Study." *Journal of Manipulative and Physiological Therapeutics* 29, no. 4 (2006): 267-74. doi:10.1016/j.jmpt.2006.03.010.

17. Weigel, Paula A.Mm., Jason M. Hockenberry, and Fredric D. Wolinsky. "Chiropractic Use in the Medicare Population: Prevalence, Patterns, and Associations With 1-Year Changes in Health and Satisfaction With Care." *Journal of Manipulative and Physiological Therapeutics* 37, no. 8 (2014): 542-51. doi:10.1016/j.jmpt.2014.08.003.

18. Keeney, Benjamin J., Deborah Fulton-Kehoe, Judith A. Turner, Thomas M. Wickizer, Kwun Chuen Gary Chan, and Gary M. Franklin. "Early Predictors of Lumbar Spine Surgery After Occupational Back Injury." *Spine* 38, no. 11 (May 15, 2013): 953-64. doi:10.1097/brs.0b013e3182814ed5.

19. Lenoir, Magalie, Fuschia Serre, Lauriane Cantin, and Serge H. Ahmed. "Intense Sweetness Surpasses Cocaine Reward." *PLoS ONE* 2, no. 8 (August 01, 2007). doi:10.1371/journal.pone.0000698.

20. Müller, Manfred. "Faculty of 1000 evaluation for Effects of dietary glycemic index on brain regions related to reward and craving in men." *F1000Prime*, June 26, 2013. doi:10.3410/f.718077314.793482444.

Chapter 6

1. Maron, Dina Fine. "Drug-Resistant Superbugs Kill At Least 23,000 People in the U.S. Each Year." *Scientific American Blog Network*. September 16, 2013. https://blogs.scientificamerican.com/observations/drug-resistant-superbugs-kill-at-least-23000-people-in-the-us-each-year/.

2. "Autoimmune diseases: a leading cause of death among young and middle-aged women in the United States." *American Journal of Public Health* 90, no. 9 (2000): 1463-466. doi:10.2105/ajph.90.9.1463.

3. "Antibiotic / Antimicrobial Resistance." *Centers for Disease Control and Prevention*. April 10, 2017. https://www.cdc.gov/drugresistance/threat-report-2013/index.html.

4. Walsh, Fergus. "Superbugs to kill 'more than cancer' by 2050." *BBC News*. December 11, 2014. http://www.bbc.com/news/health-30416844.

5. Walsh, S.J., L.M. Rau. "Autoimmune diseases: a leading cause of death among young and middle-aged women in the United States." *American Journal of Public Health* 90, no. 9 (2000): 1463-466. doi:10.2105/ajph.90.9.1463.

6. Buyken, A. E., J. Goletzke, G. Joslowski, A. Felbick, G. Cheng, C. Herder, and J. C. Brand-Miller. "Association between carbohydrate quality and inflammatory markers: systematic review of observational and interventional studies." *American Journal of Clinical Nutrition* 99, no. 4 (2014): 813-33. doi:10.3945/ajcn.113.074252.

7. Fleming-Dutra, Katherine E., Adam L. Hersh, Daniel J. Shapiro, Monina Bartoces, Eva A. Enns, Thomas M. File, Jonathan A. Finkelstein, Jeffrey S. Gerber, David Y. Hyun, Jeffrey A. Linder, Ruth Lynfield, David J. Margolis, Larissa S. May, Daniel Merenstein, Joshua P. Metlay, Jason G. Newland, Jay F. Piccirillo, Rebecca M. Roberts, Guillermo V. Sanchez, Katie J. Suda, Ann Thomas, Teri Moser Woo, Rachel M. Zetts, and Lauri A. Hicks. "Prevalence of Inappropriate Antibiotic Prescriptions Among US Ambulatory Care Visits, 2010-2011." *JAMA: The Journal of the American Medical Association* 315, no. 17 (2016): 1864. doi:10.1001/jama.2016.4151.

8. "Antibiotic / Antimicrobial Resistance." *Centers for Disease Control and Prevention*. April 10, 2017. https://www.cdc.gov/drugresistance/threat-report-2013/index.html.

9. Gorman, Christine, Alice Park, and Kristina Dell. "Cellular Inflammation: The Silent Killer." *Inflammation Research Foundation*. http://www.inflammationresearchfoundation.org/inflammation-science/inflammation-details/time-cellular-inflammation-article/.

10. Noreen, Eric E., Michael J. Sass, Megan L. Crowe, Vanessa A. Pabon, Josef Brandauer, and Lindsay K. Averill. "Effects of supplemental fish oil on resting metabolic rate, body composition, and salivary cortisol in healthy adults." *Journal of the International Society of Sports Nutrition* 7, no. 1 (October 2010): 31. doi:10.1186/1550-2783-7-31.

11. Serhan, Charles N. "Pro-resolving lipid mediators are leads for resolution physiology." *Nature* 510, no. 7503 (2014): 92-101. doi:10.1038/nature13479.

12. Spite, Matthew, Joan Clària, and Charles N. Serhan. "Resolvins, Specialized Proresolving Lipid Mediators, and Their Potential Roles in Metabolic Diseases." *Cell Metabolism* 19, no. 1 (2014): 21-36. doi:10.1016/j.cmet.2013.10.006.

13. Recchiuti, Antonio. "Immunoresolving Lipid Mediators and Resolution of Inflammation in Aging." *Journal of Gerontology & Geriatric Research* 03, no. 02 (2014). doi:10.4172/2167-7182.1000151.

14. Besedovsky, Luciana, and Jan Born. "Sleep, Don't Sneeze: Longer Sleep Reduces the Risk of Catching a Cold." *Sleep* 38, no. 9 (2015): 1341-342. doi:10.5665/sleep.4958.

15. Whiteman, Honor. "Poor sleep habits increase weight gain for adults with genetic obesity risk." *Medical News Today.* March 03, 2017. http://www.medicalnewstoday.com/articles/316186.php.

16. Celis-Morales, Carlos, Donald M. Lyall, Yibing Guo, Lewis Steell, Daniel Llanas, Joey Ward, Daniel F. Mackay, Stephany M. Biello, Mark Es Bailey, Jill P. Pell, and Jason Mr Gill. "Sleep characteristics modify the association of genetic predisposition with obesity and anthropometric measurements in 119,679 UK Biobank participants." *The American Journal of Clinical Nutrition* 105, no. 4 (2017): 980-90. doi:10.3945/ajcn.116.147231.

17. Khatib, H. K Al, S. V. Harding, J. Darzi, and G. K. Pot. "The effects of partial sleep deprivation on energy balance: a systematic review and meta-analysis." *European Journal of Clinical Nutrition* 71, no. 5 (2016): 614-24. doi:10.1038/ejcn.2016.201.

18. Kripke, Daniel F., MD. "Sleeping Pills Could Shorten Your Life." *The Dark Side of Sleeping Pills.* Accessed August 08, 2017. http://www.darksideofsleepingpills.com/.

19. Ansorge, Rick. "Enzyme Pill: A Game Changer for Gluten-Sensitive People?" *Newsmax.* May 29, 2017. http://www.newsmax.com/Health/Headline/gluten-free-celiac-enzyme/2017/05/25/id/792417/.

Endnotes

Chapter 7

1. "If Atrazine Harms Frogs and Rats, What Is It Doing to Children?" *Mercola.com.* November 12, 2016. http://articles.mercola.com/sites/articles/archive/2016/11/12/atrazine-herbicide-effects.aspx.
2. Hayes, Dr. Tyrone B., PhD. "Atrazinelovers home page." *Atrazinelovers.* http://atrazinelovers.com/.
3. Trasande, Leonardo, R. Thomas Zoeller, Ulla Hass, Andreas Kortenkamp, Philippe Grandjean, John Peterson Myers, Joseph Digangi, Martine Bellanger, Russ Hauser, Juliette Legler, Niels E. Skakkebaek, and Jerrold J. Heindel. "Estimating Burden and Disease Costs of Exposure to Endocrine-Disrupting Chemicals in the European Union." *The Journal of Clinical Endocrinology & Metabolism* 100, no. 4 (2015): 1245-255. doi:10.1210/jc.2014-4324.
4. "National Report on Human Exposure to Environmental Chemicals." *Centers for Disease Control and Prevention.* April 14, 2017. Accessed August 08, 2017. https://www.cdc.gov/exposurereport/index.html.
5. "Body Burden: The Pollution in Newborns." *Environmental Working Group.* July 14, 2005. http://www.ewg.org/research/body-burden-pollution-newborns#.
6. Trasande, Leonardo, Teresa M. Attina, and Jan Blustein. "Association Between Urinary Bisphenol A Concentration and Obesity Prevalence in Children and Adolescents." *JAMA: The Journal of the American Medical Association* 308, no. 11 (2012): 1113. doi:10.1001/2012.jama.11461.
7. Jeng, Hueiwang Anna. "Exposure to Endocrine Disrupting Chemicals and Male Reproductive Health." *Frontiers in Public Health* 2 (2014). doi:10.3389/fpubh.2014.00055.

    Meeker, John D., and Kelly K. Ferguson. "Urinary Phthalate Metabolites Are Associated With Decreased Serum Testosterone in Men, Women, and Children From NHANES 2011–2012." *The Journal of Clinical Endocrinology & Metabolism* 99, no. 11 (2014): 4346-352. doi:10.1210/jc.2014-2555.
8. Sample, Ian. "Phthalates risk damaging children's IQs in the womb, US researchers suggest." *The Guardian.* December 10, 2014. https://www.theguardian.com/lifeandstyle/2014/dec/10/phthalates-damage-childrens-iqs-womb-plastic-chemicals.
9. Braun, Joseph M., Sheela Sathyanarayana, and Russ Hauser. "Phthalate exposure and children's health." *Pediatrics* 25, no. 2 (2013): 247-54. doi:10.1097/mop.0b013e32835e1eb6.

10. Pirmohamed, M. "Adverse drug reactions as cause of admission to hospital: prospective analysis of 18 820 patients." *BMJ* 329, no. 7456 (2004): 15-19. doi:10.1136/bmj.329.7456.15.
11. "Deadly NSAIDS." *American Nutrition Association*. Accessed August 08, 2017. http://americannutritionassociation.org/newsletter/deadly-nsaids.
12. Masuoka, Howard C., and Naga Chalasani. "Nonalcoholic fatty liver disease: an emerging threat to obese and diabetic individuals." *Annals of the New York Academy of Sciences* 1281, no. 1 (2013): 106-22. doi:10.1111/nyas.12016.
13. Hazlehurst, Jonathan M., Conor Woods, Thomas Marjot, Jeremy F. Cobbold, and Jeremy W. Tomlinson. "Non-alcoholic fatty liver disease and diabetes." *Metabolism* 65, no. 8 (2016): 1096-108. doi:10.1016/j.metabol.2016.01.001.
14. Zezos, Petros. "Liver transplantation and non-alcoholic fatty liver disease." *World Journal of Gastroenterology* 20, no. 42 (November 2014): 15532. doi:10.3748/wjg.v20.i42.15532.
15. Vilar-Gomez, Eduardo, Yadina Martinez-Perez, Luis Calzadilla-Bertot, Ana Torres-Gonzalez, Bienvenido Gra-Oramas, Licet Gonzalez-Fabian, Scott L. Friedman, Moises Diago, and Manuel Romero-Gomez. "Weight Loss Through Lifestyle Modification Significantly Reduces Features of Nonalcoholic Steatohepatitis." *Gastroenterology* 149, no. 2 (2015). doi:10.1053/j.gastro.2015.04.005.
16. Axe, Josh, DNM, DC, CNS, and Eric Zielinski. "Cruciferous Vegetables: Cancer Killer or Thyroid Killers?" *Dr. Axe*. June 21, 2017. https://draxe.com/cruciferous-vegetables-cancer-thyroid/.
17. "5 Drugs You May Need to Avoid or Adjust if You Have Kidney Disease." *The National Kidney Foundation*. May 17, 2017. https://www.kidney.org/atoz/content/5-drugs-you-may-need-avoid-or-adjust-if-you-have-kidney-disease.
18. "Chronic Dehydration More Common Than You Think." *CBS Miami*. Accessed August 09, 2017. http://miami.cbslocal.com/2013/07/02/chronic-dehydration-more-common-than-you-think/.
19. Stöppler, Melissa Conrad, MD. "Cloudy Urine: Check Your Symptoms and Signs." *MedicineNet*. August 09, 2017. http://www.medicinenet.com/cloudy_urine/symptoms.htm.
20. Ebeling, Paul. "Big Pharma's Drugs in Our Water Supply, A Big Problem." *Live Trading News*. May 22, 2016. http://www.livetrading-news.com/big-pharma-drugs-water-supply-big-problem-5271.html#.

21. Parretti, Helen M., Paul Aveyard, Andrew Blannin, Susan J. Clifford, Sarah J. Coleman, Andrea Roalfe, and Amanda J. Daley. "Efficacy of water preloading before main meals as a strategy for weight loss in primary care patients with obesity: RCT." *Obesity* 23, no. 9 (2015): 1785-791. doi:10.1002/oby.21167.

22. Park, Yikyung, Amy F. Subar, Albert Hollenbeck, and Arthur Schatzkin. "Dietary Fiber Intake and Mortality in the NIH-AARP Diet and Health Study." *Archives of Internal Medicine* 171, no. 12 (2011). doi:10.1001/archinternmed.2011.18.

23. "Small increase in energy investment could cut premature deaths from air pollution in half by 2040, says new IEA report." *International Energy Agency.* June 27, 2016. https://www.iea.org/newsroom/news/2016/june/energy-and-air-pollution.html.

24. "The Inside Story: A Guide to Indoor Air Quality." *EPA.* February 28, 2017. https://www.epa.gov/indoor-air-quality-iaq/inside-story-guide-indoor-air-quality.

25. "Practical elements." *Buteyko: A to Z.* http://www.buteyko.com/practical/elements/index_elements.html.

26. "20 Houseplants That Remove Airborne Toxins From Your Home." *EcoWatch.* June 27, 2016. https://www.ecowatch.com/20-houseplants-that-remove-airborne-toxins-from-your-home-1882083322.html.

27. Genuis, Stephen J., Detlef Birkholz, Ilia Rodushkin, and Sanjay Beesoon. "Blood, Urine, and Sweat (BUS) Study: Monitoring and Elimination of Bioaccumulated Toxic Elements." *Archives of Environmental Contamination and Toxicology* 61, no. 2 (2010): 344-57. doi:10.1007/s00244-010-9611-5.